Carolyn's Story

"We must accept finite disappointment but we must never lose infinite hope."
Dr. Martin Luther King, Sr.

A true story of Postpartum Depression

Copyright 2006 by Carol S. Harcarik

All rights reserved. No part of this book may be used or reproduced in any manner without written permission from the publisher and the author, except in the case of brief quotations embodied in critical articles and reviews.

Registered with the Library of Congress, Copyright Office, September, 2006

Published by Hartington Press,
N6638 Shorewood Hills Road
Lake Mills, WI 53551
Email: hartingtonpress@aol.com

Hartington
Press
TM

Dedication

To my husband, Joe, for his unwavering support, his loving assurance and constant encouragement in the writing of this book. Also, to my four children, for their inspiration, love, strength, courage, integrity, creativity, and even tech support, which gave me the confidence that I could do this, and I did!

Table of Contents

Acknowledgements..6

Foreword..7

Prologue...8

Chapter 1 - Who is the Real Carolyn?...9

Chapter 2 - The Joyous Birth of Zachary James.........................20

Chapter 3 - It is Beginning to Sound Like PPD..........................27

Chapter 4 - Life Becomes a Nightmare.......................................36

Chapter 5 - Situation Becomes Grave...47

Chapter 6 - Electric Shock Treatments..52

Chapter 7 - ECTs are a "Living Hell"...58

Chapter 8 - Caregivers Exhausted...73

Chapter 9 - Appeared ECTs Failed...81

Chapter 10 - Carolyn Arrives at Mayo Clinic.............................90

Chapter 11 - Mayo Clinic -- Medical Breakthrough...................98

Chapter 12 - Cognitive Behavior Therapy................................. 104

Chapter 13 - Did the ECTs Work?...113

Chapter 14 - Carolyn Gets Her Life Back.................................119

Chapter 15 - They finally become a Family...............................129

Table of Contents

Epilogue..138

Family Pictures..142-146

Keys to Survival...147

Note from Author..148

PPD Symptoms..149

Comments from Author......................................150-151

References..152

Book Offer..153

About Author...154

Acknowledgements

Overwhelming gratitude to Carolyn, her family, and nanny for their help in writing this book. They were all most patient with me. Carolyn was a constant support; always supplying as much information as she could, and setting up the appointments for the interviews at Mayo Clinic.

Carolyn had an extensive memory loss following the birth of her son, Zachary, so the story surrounding the birth was told to me through interviews with her mother, Mary-Jane, her husband, Demian, and Zachary's nanny, Betty. I did interview Carolyn, after her memory returned, and she gave me background information. Also, thanks to Jessica Hosszu, Carolyn's dear friend, for her telephone interview.

Interview with David Mrazek, M.D., Chair, Mayo Clinic Department of Psychiatry and Psychology.

Interview with Renato D. Alarcon, M.D., Medical Director, Mayo Clinic Psychiatry and Psychology Treatment Center and Mood Disorders Unit. Dr. Alarcon was the psychiatrist who led Carolyn's treatment team and saw her on a daily basis when she was at the Mayo Clinic.

Interview with Grant Bauer, a licensed, independent, Clinical Social Worker, Mayo Clinic Department of Psychiatry and Psychology. Grant worked directly with Carolyn on her medical team while she was a patient at Mayo Clinic.

Interview with Roseanne Clark, Ph.D., Director Parent-Infant and Early Childhood Clinic and UW Postpartum Depression Treatment Program, Department of Psychiatry, University of Wisconsin School of Medicine and Public Health, Madison, WI Dr. Clark never met or treated Carolyn. Her interview provided important background information to the author on Postpartum Depression.

Special thanks to Kerry Feuerman, a dear friend and mentor to Carolyn. Kerry is responsible for our fabulous title: "Mommies Cry, Too! A Painful and Triumphant Story of Postpartum Depression."

Special thanks to Rita Bill and Julie Clark, my dear friends, for their moral and editing support.

Foreword

Carolyn's courage allows us to know her tragic story so that others will become familiar with the facts, consequences and treatments of the mental disorder called postpartum depression (PPD), which in some cases can be horrific. Many more women need to be aware of the serious ramifications of overlooking PPD's symptoms and to help other women reach beyond the stigma toward acceptance of its very existence. Only then will we, as a society, begin to recognize this illness for what it is and get help in managing PPD before it can cause damage to its victim and the victim's family.

It is estimated PPD affects 15 - 20 percent of new mothers. A small percentage will get the new-baby blues and the rest will have PPD with varying degrees of severity. One in 1,000 will get PPD psychosis. Untreated, severe PPD can be a fatal illness.

The cause of PPD is not fully known. What is known is that there is usually a *history of depression* in the victim's family and the *hormonal adjustment* that happens normally after birth appears to negatively affect people who get PPD. Many women do not realize that their bodies have high levels of estrogen prior to giving birth and that immediately after birth the estrogen level drops dramatically. This can cause a *biochemical change* in brain function. There also appears to be a definite link to specific *personality traits* in PPD sufferers.

In the story that follows, Carolyn was affected by all four known causes of PPD, and she, also, had some extenuating life circumstances that may have increased the severity of her PPD.

Prologue by Carolyn

The first three months of my baby's life are completely erased from my memory. I don't remember going into labor, the birth, bringing him home from the hospital or even his early doctor's appointments. As I now contemplate the enormity of that statement, I wonder if I even want the memories to come back. According to anyone who was a part of my life at that time, it was absolute hell on earth for me and everyone else involved. But what will happen one day when my son asks me, "Mommy, what happened on the day I was born?" or, "What was it like when you brought me home from the hospital?" What will I say? "Sorry, son, I don't remember, ask your father"? Will he think that I didn't love him enough to remember such an important time in his life? Will he be able to understand what happened to me? Do I even understand what happened to me? Even now, after several months of feeling much like my old self, I don't quite think that I do.

Everyone says the memories will come back, that over time and with exposure I will begin to be able to put the pieces back together. At least the important ones, like the day he was born and the time we spent together before postpartum depression drew me into its black hole of despair. For now, I'll have to tell my story as others have told it to me. I need to do this so I can begin to heal and understand what happened to me, but also to continue to try to chip away at the stigma that is associated with mental illness. What few people understand is that postpartum depression is a real illness, not something that people can simply "snap out of" or "pull themselves up by their bootstraps" and get over. It is about hormones and brain chemistry, much of it too complicated for me to ever understand, but a real illness nonetheless. No one would whisper behind closed doors if I had been diagnosed with cancer after my son's birth. I hope one day, the same can be said about postpartum depression and all other mental illnesses.

Chapter 1

Who is the Real Carolyn?

Carolyn has a complete personality change

Carolyn loses her memory from the time her son, Zachary, is born, until three to four months later when she experiences an awakening and finds her awareness returning. She has this strange realization that she has become a different person. After taking her morning shower, she dressed and was brushing her teeth when she noticed the person she was looking at in the mirror was a bit overweight and was not a blonde but a brunette. Carolyn thought to herself, "It feels like I just woke up and everything is different. It feels eerie and I feel sorta disconnected and detached." She looked in the mirror at herself again and said, "Oh my goodness, I really gained weight. How did this happen? This is really weird." Then she just went on with the day somewhat confused.

The lack of strong feelings for such an abrupt change was

not normal for Carolyn. Her usual inquisitiveness had disappeared and she remembers passively accepting the situation. She said, "I wasn't sad, angry, or curious, just confused. I did not ask anyone in my immediate family what happened to me, I just seemed to be distracted and somewhat dazed by it all."

She had gained a little weight because of the medication she was on for postpartum depression and her hair had started to change from blonde to brown during her pregnancy. Because of her three-month memory loss and the horrible ordeal she had been through, she really <u>was</u> looking at a very different person.

Carolyn's mother, Mary-Jane, her husband, Demian, and Zachary's nanny, Betty, needed to fill in for her, the three-month segment of her life that had been erased. They all wondered how they were going to handle this delicate situation.

Mary-Jane pondered, "How can anyone describe to someone else the birth of their child, and those precious early months of life when your baby needs you so much because he is so vulnerable, tiny, sweet, and precious. This is almost an impossible task for anyone. I've never heard of this type of loss -- it's so profound and painful to comprehend. How will I ever get her to understand all of this?"

Mary-Jane tried her best to fill in all the details by telling Carolyn about her normal birth and delivery and the great excitement, involving the entire family, that followed Zachary's birth. At the same time, she expressed great sorrow, that Carolyn could not remember anything about this important event in her life. Mary-Jane also had to tell her about the hell they had all been through including the electric shock treatments (electroconvulsive therapy or ECT) she had, how difficult this time had been for all of them and how concerned they had been for her. She had been suicidal and had experienced a complete personality change.

Demian said to Carolyn, "You had a 'perfect storm.' At least that's my theory. Along with your sunny, giving spirit, the in-charge perfectionist side of your personality sometimes made you somewhat compulsive -- and remember when you took the birth control pill, we noticed that your sensitivity to estrogen caused your mood to be rather mercurial, quiet one day and excitable and dramatic the next day. But the final blow was your coping strategy for living your life that has always benefited you and made you the wonderful person you are; but in this situation it failed you. You know what your motto has always been: Don't spend time worrying about something until something happens that you really need to worry about. These three things collided and made a perfect storm. It's really so unfair that this happened to you. You are the nicest person I know."

Betty was Zachary's nanny, and had also taken care of Carolyn during her PPD. She had become a "Guardian Angel" to all the family. Betty said, "I remember with great sadness and will never forget Carolyn's mother, Mary-Jane, saying to me, 'The Carolyn you are taking care of along with Zachary is not really my daughter, she is a totally different person.'" Betty added, "That just blew my mind and I did not know what to expect."

What was Carolyn like before Zachary's birth?

Carolyn, by nature, is an inquisitive person, highly intelligent, achievement-oriented and fun-loving. Her physical beauty is evident, along with her gregarious nature.

Her husband described her as one of the most positive people he has ever met. He said, "She is a very confident person with a huge heart, an indomitable will, highly organized and can do anything if she puts her mind to it." He added, "She is just fantastic."

Carolyn's father, Mike, complimented her by saying, "She has always had a stunning personality, very sociable, energetic, with obvious leadership qualities that enable her to draw people to her like a magnet. She actually considers herself a 'type A' personality, but she's really more than that."

Carolyn's younger years

Carolyn grew up with her younger brother and two loving parents, and was surrounded by a wonderful extended family. She describes her childhood as fun-filled and happy with parents who always challenged her, but never pressured her.

Her grandmother was a central figure in the early years of her life and her personality was a lot like Carolyn's -- fun-loving and gregarious. Her grandmother doted on her and they spent many happy times together. When Carolyn was about six years old her grandmother died, and this was a sad time for her in an otherwise happy childhood.

Mommies Cry Too

Carolyn excelled academically and skipped fourth grade. Her classmates in fifth grade intimidated her by insisting she wouldn't be able to do the work; but her "indomitable will" clicked in and proved them wrong. But this experience would have an effect on her attitude toward her academic life. She tended to keep the intellectual side of her personality private in return for being popular and fun. She continued to excel academically, but she never spoke to any of her friends about her grades. Even as a child she was a very structured, motivated and organized individual.

In high school, she was popular, and had a few boyfriends, plus her share of the common high school problems. Her parents knew they were dealing with a bright, strong-willed personality and used their parental wisdom to keep her on the right track.

To round out her education Carolyn went to France for a year after high school and then went on to college. She studied hard and continued to excel academically. She made many friends at college and met her lifelong best friend, Jess, there.

Carolyn sighed as she said, "My four years at college are

like a blur in my life. I never realized that life could be so full of fun and carefree."

Carolyn enters life in the real world

After graduating from college with a B.A. in psychology Carolyn was hired as a marketing account manager and successfully managed advertising for a national chain of stores. Carolyn said, "The first day on the job I met Demian, a warm, gentle, articulate man with the most amazing, expressive brown eyes I had ever seen. He became the love of my life and I knew immediately upon meeting him that this was the man I was going to marry! Eventually, that is exactly what happened. He turned out to be the perfect balance and complement to me -- calm to my excitable, steady to my highs and lows. He loved me unconditionally from the beginning."

After a few years of marriage, Carolyn and Demian moved to Richmond, Virginia, a lovely genteel southern city where they were both hired by the same advertising firm. They purchased a home and fell in love with southern life and culture. For the next two years they settled into their new jobs and toured the surrounding area. Carolyn remembers this

Mommies Cry Too

time of their marriage as very special, because they spent so much time together just having fun and enjoying each other's company.

They made many new friends and began to think about starting a family. She said, "Our lives, though wonderful, were very self-involved and we felt like we wanted something more and maybe that something more would be a baby. We always knew we wanted children. I was 28 years old and the time seemed right, so I stopped taking birth control pills and hoped for the best."

Carolyn shares the following story: "It so happened that around this time, Hurricane Isabel came up the Atlantic coast. There were hurricane warnings all over town, so Demian purchased a lot of extra supplies and we hunkered down for the big storm. Soon after the hurricane hit, the power went out, and it was like we were the only two people in the world and it created a crazy romantic atmosphere that actually lasted for several days. It was kinda wonderful, really. And, yes, about a month later we discovered we were pregnant, and considered ourselves so fortunate to get pregnant so easily. It was absolutely thrilling to think that we were going to become a real family!"

Carolyn could hardly wait to tell her mom about the baby. They had always had a strong relationship and she was eager to share their news. She proudly said, "My mom is my best friend. We talk every day. In my life, it has never seemed as if decisions were quite final until she said they were good decisions. We also are very comfortable around each other and love to discuss anything and everything. Having her there after the birth would center me. She is so sensible and tremendously strong."

So, with great enthusiasm and creativity, Carolyn came up with a cute little scheme to tell both sets of grandparents the news. She said, "We sent them birthday party invitations and indicated it was a party for their grandchild and the date of the party was my due date. It was a wonderful way to break the news and since it would be the first grandchild for both sets of grandparents, they were all hysterical with excitement."

Demian and Carolyn had fun getting ready for the baby by redoing an upstairs room in their home. They knew the baby was a boy and had picked out the name Zachary James. They would sit in Zachary's room together and it was so perfect with the crib, dresser and all the other things a baby needs. The only thing missing was a baby, and it was impossible to comprehend that it was really happening. Carolyn said, "We used to sit in there and try to imagine what he would be like, what qualities of the other we hoped he would have. Would he eat and sleep well? How much would we love him, how would he change our lives? We could never have imagined the love we would feel. It surpassed all of our hopes and dreams."

Carolyn had a relatively normal pregnancy which included a bout with morning sickness in her first trimester. In her last trimester, however, she did have a worrisome experience. During one of her regular checkups, her ob-gyn doctor discovered she had dysplasia (precancerous) cells on her cervix. The doctor told Carolyn that nothing could be done about them until after the baby was born. "After your six-week checkup we'll decide on a time when we can remove them," she said. "Don't worry about this because it's not cancer it's pre-cancer, and once they are removed you can just forget about it."

Despite her doctor's reassurance, this must have caused some anxious moments for Carolyn. However, she stuck to her motto and decided not to worry about it until she really had something to worry about. She did notice, however, that she would often feel anxious about unimportant incidents and sometimes felt tense and oversensitive. She figured, "I'm pregnant, that explains it."

Overall, Carolyn was healthy and strong throughout her pregnancy and like all expectant mothers, all she hoped for was a healthy baby. She and Demian were excited and full of anticipation to meet Zachary, to know him and to love him.

Chapter 2

The Joyous Birth of Zachary James

A joyous birth quickly unfolds into a tragic story

Zachary was born on Monday, May 17, 2004 at 3:07 p.m and weighed in at 8 lbs. 8 oz. Demian and Carolyn were overjoyed with their little guy and as proud as they could be. He was equally welcomed by his maternal grandparents, Mary-Jane and Mike, and his paternal grandparents, Lois and Jim. Carolyn had come through the delivery well and there were no complications for her or Zachary.

There were, however, a few problems. Zachary's pediatrician discovered what appeared to be an insignificant birth defect affecting his frenulum. This birth defect causes the tissue that attaches the tongue to the bottom of the mouth to be abnormally short (commonly known as tongue-tie). The pediatrician clipped the tissue which fixed the problem. Zachary had jaundice, as well, which is not uncommon in newborns and is caused when there is a higher-than-normal amount of bilirubin in the blood -- a byproduct of decomposing red blood cells normally excreted by the liver. The pediatrician told Carolyn that the best way to get rid of jaundice is to encourage the baby to nurse as much as possible because that would help lower the bilirubin levels.

So, on the Wednesday after his birth, Demian and Carolyn brought home their beautiful new baby boy. It was all very exciting! The plan was that Mary-Jane would stay for a few weeks to help them out. But little did they know that a nightmare was about to unfold.

Almost immediately, something seems amiss

Demian recalls that he was a little concerned about the expression Carolyn had on her face while she was holding the baby for the first time after he was born. He said, "Her look was not an excited 'WOW,' but rather she looked mystified, confused and even worried." He added, "Here I was crying for joy because Zachary was holding my finger and it seemed strange to me that Carolyn looked so serious. I guessed she was feeling a bit awe-struck with the responsibility of raising a child."

Zachary rejects the breast

Only two days after entering the world, Zachary made it quite clear he did not want to breast-feed. "He screamed when put to the breast and would not latch on," Carolyn's mother recalled. "Zachary's reaction created a difficult dilemma for Carolyn. She was conscientious about doing the best for her baby and planned on breast-feeding, but Zachary refused to cooperate and she never expected to be rejected in this way." Dr. Alarcon, a psychiatrist at Mayo Clinic who would later treat Carolyn for PPD, said, "The rejection of the breast, for a person with Carolyn's personality, was particularly painful."

Mary-Jane said, "Carolyn had received a lot of instruction on breast-feeding at the hospital and insisted on continuing to try. Zachary was just as insistent with his constant refusals. All three of us made the decision for Carolyn to pump breast milk, so Demian and I could help with the feedings. We were also concerned because we remembered the statement by the pediatrician. "The best way to get rid of jaundice is for Zachary to be well-fed." We were concerned he was not getting enough to eat and we felt this was the best alternative. The hospital had given Carolyn some formula when she left, so she starting pumping breast milk and mixing it with the formula, hoping she would eventually be able to convince Zachary to take over on the breast." Mary-Jane added, "That seemed unlikely to me because he appeared to be very fond of the bottle."

Carolyn took Zachary back and forth to the lactation specialist at her ob-gyn's office, but they were equally unsuccessful in getting him to latch on. Carolyn and Demian agonized over this dilemma. They knew it was better to breast-feed and they did not like giving up. For Carolyn, things were getting out of control.

Roseanne Clark, Ph.D., Director, Postpartum Depression Treatment Program, University of Wisconsin School of Medicine and Public Health, said, "When a woman becomes a new mother, and she has perfectionistic tendencies, she may view her baby's difficulty with breast-feeding as a rejection of her or a failure on her part."

Carolyn feels panicky and overwhelmed

Carolyn's mother said, "At this point, the end result of the breast-feeding problem was that Carolyn and the baby had little calm time together because she was always trying to breast-feed him and that would lead to his screaming rejection. Zachary seemed quite happy with the bottle, and it was clear to me he had made his decision. He did not want the breast and appeared quite satisfied with the way things were going."

According to Mary-Jane, Zachary's rejection of the breast seemed to be the catalyst that started panicky feelings in Carolyn. On top of that, she was a bit frantic about getting enough food in him so that he would get rid of the jaundice. Consequently, she was getting very little sleep and her stress level was rising.

Demian mentioned to Carolyn that his parents wanted to visit the new baby over the weekend. Carolyn quickly suggested, "Please tell them not to come because we are trying to resolve the breast-feeding problem and I can't handle house guests at this particular time." She thought to herself, "I just can't seem to get control of this situation."

Demian concluded this was new-mom jitters and told his parents to come ahead. So the in-laws arrived for their weekend visit. At about the same time, it was clear that the jaundice was not clearing up. Demian was concerned, so he called the pediatrician's office. The pediatrician said the quickest and easiest way to get rid of jaundice is to put the baby under special lights for a specified time each day, so he immediately had the hospital send over the lights. But Carolyn was thinking, "Things are even more out of control; the baby won't breast-feed and the jaundice is not getting better."

Mary-Jane anxiously pointed out, "The baby was only a few days old and we were quickly trying to balance a number of problems. The in-laws were visiting, Zachary's jaundice was not improving, we were afraid he was not getting enough to eat and he had refused the breast. Carolyn had very little sleep, her panicky feelings were increasing, she was feeling intensely overwhelmed and was starting to feel that something was wrong with her. She was confused by all this and couldn't understand what was happening to her.

Carolyn called her friends to see if these kinds of feelings happened to them when they had their babies. After she talked to them, she said to her mom, "I don't seem to be having the same feelings as my friends did." Those conversations just made her feelings of despair increase; it was only the Sunday after Zachary's birth, not even a week, and Carolyn appeared panic-stricken and very overwhelmed.

What was wrong with Carolyn? Was it PPD?

Dr. Alarcon, from Mayo Clinic, later described, "There are four components to PPD. There is usually a genetic predisposition to depression, biochemical malfunctions in the brain affecting the central nervous system, problems with hormone levels, and specific personality traits. PPD is really clinical depression with a few differences. The differences are that it happens following birth and has a hormonal component. Otherwise, the treatment is, in general terms, the same as it is for clinical depression. The trigger is usually the birth."

Meanwhile, Demian and Mary-Jane sensed something was very wrong but didn't know what. In the back of their minds they were both dreading that maybe this was PPD.

Chapter 3

It's Beginning to sound like PPD

Carolyn has symptoms of PPD

Mary-Jane realized she was scheduled to go home in about a week but it was becoming apparent that was not going to happen. Zachary was just about a week old and both she and Demian decided they were dealing with something unusual. They found a list of symptoms for postpartum depression and were shocked as they went down the list and checked off every one of them, because they all related to Carolyn's current behavior. Also they both remembered Carolyn's sensitivity to estrogen when she was on the birth control pill. The information they were reading on the symptoms of PPD stated that the dramatic drop in estrogen following birth played a part in the disorder. (See page 149 for a list of the symptoms of PPD.)

Dr. Clark states, "Postpartum depression often results from a complex interaction of biological and psychosocial factors. Childbirth can be a time of major psychological and interpersonal adjustment."

So the Monday following the birth, Demian and Mary-Jane called the ob-gyn doctor and suggested that perhaps Carolyn had PPD. When they spoke with the doctor she said, "I doubt this is PPD, it's more likely to be sleep deprivation. Get someone to take over the night feedings, see if you can get her to take an afternoon nap and then she can get caught up on her sleep." So Demian took the evening feeding and Mary-Jane took over the night feedings. Fortunately, they had a good baby who was waking up only a few times a night and who eagerly took his bottle and went right back to sleep afterward.

They continued to be concerned, however, because they were noticing strange changes in Carolyn's behavior. She was not her inquisitive self, no longer quick on the uptake or full of curiosity. She seemed dazed, 'kinda' out of it', too compliant. She would make comments like, "What made me think I could do this? I'm not the mother type, I'm just not capable. This is too hard. I've made a big mistake. This is incredibly life-changing and I don't want to be here." She seemed so flustered with the daily routine that the smallest pressures seem to knock her off kilter. This wasn't normal or at all like her. She would say, "Somebody else has to take care of Zachary, I can't handle this."

Her mother said, "Carolyn never focused on hurting the baby, but just kept saying, 'This is too much work,' when she really wasn't doing that much work. She found bathing Zachary to be very scary and couldn't see how she was going to fit it into the day's schedule. She wasn't making sense." Mary-Jane and Demian wanted to say to her, "Hey, just get over this," but they were sensing something serious was going on. It would have been easy to overlook her behavior, but Mary-Jane knew her daughter and knew something was beginning to appear very wrong. Demian was also getting rather alarmed.

One evening, Carolyn and her mother were feeding Zachary, and Carolyn made the following shocking statement: "I'm going to have to give Zachary up for adoption." She added, "Having this baby was a mistake." Horrified, Mary-Jane said, "Putting Zachary up for adoption is not going to happen, Demian would not agree to this and neither would Dad or I, and that's all there is to it. You wanted this baby and he is not leaving this house. This baby is not going anywhere." Carolyn was not happy with that response and Mary-Jane stared at her in complete disbelief. Both she and Demian tried to reason with her to no avail. They were anguished by what she had said and felt their concern growing.

Dramatic lifestyle change

Carolyn had worked at her marketing job right up to the day before she went into labor. She had made dramatic changes in her lifestyle in only a matter of a few days, and combined with her personality traits, this may have contributed to her PPD. Dr. Clark who never met Carolyn, described the losses a woman who leaves a high-power position may experience: "Women with careers may experience significant lifestyle changes when they leave their jobs to become a mother. Daily tasks such as feeding her baby, diaper-changing and laundry can feel unending. There is also the loss of sleep and loss of feeling in control and because of the time and energy demands of childcare, a woman may experience a loss of intimacy with her partner. In addition, there is the loss of adult relationships at work. The loss of a paycheck may also make a woman feel more dependent and many professional women have never been aware of their dependency needs. The responsibilities of motherhood can be over-whelming. This can, for some women, be a very debilitating experience that may contribute to low self esteem and guilt about not being the perfect mother."

Carolyn is put on medication for PPD

In exasperation Mary-Jane said, "The plan for Carolyn to get more sleep had sounded like a good idea, but it turned out she could not seem to sleep at all." She said Carolyn would go to her room and not be able to sleep and then be afraid to come downstairs because she would have to take care of the baby. "So, she was basically up in her room hiding. Once, when I went to check on her I discovered the situation. I tried to calm her down by talking to her calmly and suggested she try some deep breathing techniques. Nothing worked! I could not calm her down and she could not calm herself down. I called the doctor back and she put Carolyn on the antidepressant Zoloft immediately. Zoloft is considered the best treatment for PPD because it will not harm the baby through the breast milk and Carolyn was still pumping breast milk and Zachary was getting a mixture of formula and breast milk."

Mommies Cry Too

Her mother asked Carolyn if the Zoloft was helping. Carolyn tried to analyze her feelings by saying, "I may be depressed, but this anxiety makes my heart race. I feel so overwhelmed and panicky that I don't want to leave the house." She added, "There seems to be something more going on here."

Carolyn is able to articulate her feelings

Fortunately, Carolyn was always analytical and it seemed that she retained this ability to analyze her feelings even under these difficult circumstances. She also was vocal and honest about her feelings and direct about saying, "I don't want this baby." Her statements were so hurtful to her mother and they made her angry with Carolyn; but it was important that she voiced her feelings and got them out even though it was hard for her loved ones to hear. Often women will keep these kinds of negative feelings bottled up inside because they know having a baby is supposed to be a happy time and they are afraid to let anyone else know how they feel. Then their guilt, shame and humiliation, because they don't want their babies, will compound the problem or make the problem even worse.

Mary-Jane said, "Carolyn's statements were a guide or a gauge to me as to what step to take next. Her ability to verbalize her feelings helped me to make decisions and to decide what was working and what wasn't. It also helped me to know if we were in a crisis or should we wait it out. Even though her words were often tough to take, in the end they were critical."

An anti-anxiety medication is prescribed

Because Carolyn was expressing constant feelings of anxiety, her mother called the doctor again and she prescribed an anti-anxiety medication called Ativan. The doctor cautioned Mary-Jane not to let Carolyn take it on a continual basis because she could become addicted. The doctor emphasized, "Use it very carefully." Mary-Jane explained all of this information to Carolyn.

It was obvious to all of them that the anxiety and the panic were the driving force of the problem. She was panicky about everything and that appeared to be the main problem, not depression.

Carolyn did, however, make the decision not to take the

anti-anxiety medication right away. She decided that perhaps the depression was causing the anxiety, and she was afraid the addictive qualities of the medication might harm the baby through her breast milk. She stuck with the Zoloft. This was an example of Carolyn's strength. Despite her extreme anxiety and distress, Zachary's welfare and care were foremost in her mind.

Mary-Jane was becoming more concerned that Carolyn was receiving an antidepressant and had been given a prescription for anti-anxiety medication without a psychiatrist overseeing the types of medication and the dosage. She knew she had to get Carolyn to a psychiatrist. She called Carolyn's ob-gyn's office and asked for advice. They suggested she make an appointment with their therapist who worked with PPD patients. Mary-Jane took Carolyn to see the therapist and while driving to the office she noticed that Carolyn seemed a little calmer. She concluded the antidepressant must be starting to work.

Carolyn spent a lot of time with the therapist and came out with written instructions on how to help herself. Interestingly, Carolyn was already doing everything the therapist suggested: calming techniques, breathing techniques, getting enough rest, eating properly, and getting exercise. That evening when they sat down to dinner, they comforted each other by saying, "Well, we know what the problem is, we know what the solution is, and we're on the right path."

Carolyn was scheduled to see the therapist regularly, but still they needed to find a competent psychiatrist to be certain that the medication and dosage were correct.

Chapter 4

Life becomes a Nightmare

The nightmare is reality

Zachary was now two weeks old. They had a couple of fairly good days, but then the anxiety started to build up again. "One day I will never forget," Mary-Jane said. "I was sitting in the living room resting and Carolyn came downstairs from her afternoon nap. She sat down on the edge of the chair and she appeared very strange. She began moving her arms in a jerky and awkward fashion and her voice was very shaky. Then she said, 'I figured out what is wrong with me.'"

Mary-Jane said, "Really, what is it?" Carolyn said, "I've been thinking this through very carefully while I've been upstairs and I should not be here anymore. I am going to have to go away and I should never have had a baby. I don't know what made me have a baby. We didn't think it through, you know. I can't handle it, maybe Demian would

36

like to keep him but I can't cope with it anymore."

Mary-Jane looked at her daughter in shock and despair. She began to think, "She has really lost her mind. Oh, my God, what am I going to do with her?" Carolyn continued, "If I could just take my mind out of my head. It's betraying me. I've never had these kind of thoughts before. I don't understand what is happening to me." Her mother said to her, "Where are you planning to go? What would you live on and where would you work?" Carolyn said, "I don't know."

At the time, the significance of this conversation didn't register, but later Mary-Jane was shocked and terrified to realize that Carolyn was really trying to tell her that she was thinking about suicide. When she shared her suspicions with Demian, they both became frantic because this was completely out of character for Carolyn. She never backed down from a challenge and always had confidence that any problem could be fixed with perseverance and determination. Demian was very worried and scared now. He felt very discouraged and said to Mary-Jane, "We just aren't making any progress."

In desperation, Mary-Jane suggested that Carolyn take some

of the Ativan, the anti-anxiety medication. It worked almost immediately and Carolyn experienced some relief. She soon seemed less anxious and depressed. So, at this point, because of the possibility that the anti-anxiety medication could get into the breast milk, she stopped the breast pumping and reluctantly decided to bottle-feed Zachary. That didn't seem to bother him in the least. He thrived on the formula and thoroughly enjoyed his bottle.

A psychiatrist is essential

Mary-Jane knew more than ever they needed to find a psychiatrist. If she had been in her own hometown of Madison, Wisconsin, where she had lived for several years, she would have had many opportunities to seek recommendations for a competent psychiatrist. Her social circle included many doctors and their spouses; plus she had many trusted friends who would have done anything in their power to help her. Considering the medical crisis that she now found herself in, those contacts would have given her much-needed advice, comfort and direction. But, unfortunately, that was not the case; she was in Carolyn's hometown and knew no one. Carolyn, herself, had not lived there very long and did not know that many people. So, the best she could do was turn

Mommies Cry Too

to the Yellow Pages and the several area clinics listed there.

Mary-Jane reflected, "The first doctor I found couldn't see her for two months, but by that time, she would have been dead." Finally, she found a psychiatrist who appeared to be acceptable. He saw Carolyn and Mary-Jane together and said Carolyn was taking the right medication but the wrong dosage. So he raised the dosage of both, the antidepressant and the anti-anxiety medication. For a short time afterward Carolyn was a little better, but then she got worse again. They went back to see him and he said, "You know, this is very very serious and you must take it seriously and watch her carefully." Mary-Jane thought to herself, "You are not telling me anything I don't know." They carried on for another couple of weeks. Initially Carolyn was better, then worse, then she plateaued. Mary-Jane and Demian realized they weren't making any real progress. Day by day they expected her to get better but she didn't improve. Then one day the medication seemed to stop working completely, she got very panicky and anxious again and was expressing suicidal thoughts. Both Carolyn and her mother decided they needed to find another psychiatrist. So, Mary-Jane went back to the Yellow Pages to look for another one.

39

Carolyn is hospitalized

Mary-Jane found a postpartum clinic listed, she called the number and was told by the receptionist that Carolyn could not be seen until Monday. Mary-Jane screamed at her, "Carolyn is suicidal. What am I going to do?" The receptionist calmly said, "If that is the situation, you must take her to the emergency room at the hospital right away. They have a program all set up for just this type of problem and it includes a team of experts who will evaluate the situation. You need to go to the emergency room right now."

Mary-Jane called Demian immediately. When he came home Carolyn took him to another room, away from Zachary, who was now four weeks old. She whispered to him, "I don't want the baby and I don't want him to hear what I'm saying because I know babies pick up on everything. I don't want him to know how I feel. My mother thinks I should go to the emergency room. She's never asked me to do that before so I guess I better go." Demian said, "You know your mother has been calling the shots pretty well and I think you better do as she says and go to the emergency room." Carolyn was very compliant and replied meekly, "O.K."

Mommies Cry Too

Mary-Jane hurried Carolyn off to the emergency room. When the receptionist at admitting asked Carolyn why she was there, she said, "Well, I think I have postpartum depression." The receptionist was incredibly kind and then asked her if she was having thoughts of suicide and Carolyn said, "Yes." She told Carolyn that she was going to be all right and that they had a medical team set up to handle situations like this.

Carolyn asked her mother to accompany her and they met with a social worker and a psychiatrist. Carolyn told them in a very matter-of-fact manner and completely unemotional way, "I have made a bad decision and I don't want this baby. I know it upsets my mother when she hears me say this, but I just don't want the baby. I am very depressed and anxious, and I guess if my mother says I need to be here, then I need to be here." She was very non-committal.

Mary-Jane explained, "The diagnosis from the psychiatrist and social worker was that Carolyn had PPD bordering on psychosis. She was having some obsessive-compulsive thoughts, some detachment from reality, but she did not hear voices and was not hallucinating; this would have meant she had full-blown psychosis. She needed to be admitted to the hosptal for a week to get on a different medication. They put her on the antidepressant Lexapro along with an anti-anxiety medication and told her that in a week she would be feeling great and she wouldn't even recognize herself. Carolyn said, 'All right, if you think this is the right thing to do.' She never even gave a thought to who was going to take care the baby." All Mary-Jane could do was cry and say, "Oh, my God!"

"Carolyn perked up in the hospital, her verbal expressions turned around, and she started to feel pretty good," her mother recalled. Her attitude seemed improved and she said, "I still have thoughts that I don't want the baby, but I think they will go away slowly." She tried to get released in five days but the team insisted that she stay seven. They told her there's usually a relapse if a patient goes home too early

Carolyn came home on a Friday and on Saturday morning she got up in great spirits, and she and Demian went to visit some friends and even took Zachary with them. Her mother thought, "Oh, thank God, we're going to see the end of this now." Demian also thought that they had finally turned the corner. *That lasted one day!*

Mary Jane couldn't believe how quickly Carolyn returned to her very depressed and anxiety-ridden state. She kept saying, "I just don't want to be here, and I don't want this baby." Her mother said, "The next two days were absolutely terrible! Worse than before she went into the hospital. She constantly spoke of suicide."

Carolyn was upset about feeling bad again, and pointed out to her mom, "The doctor in the hospital told me that I was going to have some good days and bad days but as long as there were more good days than bad I would be making progress. He also said I might have a downturn." Mary-Jane managed to calm down and agreed with Carolyn's analysis that what they were probably experiencing was just a downturn. Yet the up and down days continued and it was difficult to judge whether she was really making progress. Some days they got though fairly well, but the mornings were never good. As the day progressed she tended to get a little better.

Mary-Jane takes Carolyn to their Florida seaside condo

After coming home from the hospital and experiencing this constant up and down emotional turmoil, Mary-Jane decided to take Carolyn to their seaside condo with the hope that maybe a change of scenery would help. Carolyn did fairly well there. She was really trying and the new medication was beginning to work so she was feeling a little better. She went for walks with her mom every day and took the baby down to the beach. Mary-Jane remembered Carolyn made her dad a cake for his birthday and showed some little signs of improvement. Zachary was starting to smile a bit and responding to her, so that was positive. Overall, it was a pretty good week. They began to think they were making progress and perhaps she would gradually get better from here on.

When they left to go back to Carolyn's home, her mother started to notice that Carolyn was getting a little panicky on the plane. Mary-Jane thought to herself, "Leaving the safety of our home seems to be causing her increased anxiety, because now she has to go back to her own home where she will be responsible for taking care of the baby." The closer they got to her home the more agitated she became. Mary-Jane tried in vain to calm her down. The next morning, when she woke up in her own bed, it was like she had never been away. She was in a horrible state again. She was depressed, suicidal and did not want the baby. Zachary was now six weeks old. Her mother could not help but be discouraged and it seemed that they just weren't getting anywhere.

Six-week checkup offers more bad news

Mary-Jane took Carolyn to her ob-gyn doctor for her six-week check-up just as she was reverting back to her very depressed and anxiety-ridden state. Mary-Jane said, "To make matters even worse, during her pregnancy Carolyn had been diagnosed with pre-cancerous cells on her cervix. She had been assured that it was not cancer, but was told at this six-week check-up, that those cells would have to be scraped off the cervix. This, of course, meant surgery, outpatient surgery, but still something we didn't need at this point in time. The ob-gyn doctor did not address the PPD. As far as she was concerned, this was a problem for the therapist or psychiatrist, not her. There was no help for us there."

It seemed to Mary-Jane their problems were mounting and when she arrived home that day she found out they had a new one. Demian had a history of extensive ear problems ever since he was a child. He had ear surgery in 1999 to remove a cholesteatoma. This type of tumor is agressive and eats away at the tissue and bone so it needs to be removed immediately."

Since they had moved to Virgina, because of his lifelong history of ear problems, Demian went for regular checkups to Johns Hopkins University Hospital. During his most recent checkup, they discovered the tumor had grown back. This condition is painless, so fortunately for him he had kept to his checkup schedule. The tumor is fast-growing, non-cancerous and was on his right eardrum and would have to be removed as soon as possible. When Mary-Jane heard this, the first thing that came to her mind was, "What else could possibly go wrong, this is unbelievable!"

Chapter 5

Situation becomes Grave

Mary-Jane faces the gravity of the situation

At this point, Mary-Jane realized Carolyn needed outpatient surgery, although she was still depressed and suicidal. The baby was almost two months old and there seemed to be no end in sight to the PPD; and to top it all off, Demian now needed surgery. There really had been no relief. She also realized that she was not going to get home anytime soon. She thought, "We are not getting anywhere, and this is already July." She called the psychiatrist, who changed the medication from Lexapro to Paxil. Mary-Jane followed through on the change of medication but was losing confidence that this was going to help. She was beginning to realize she was going to need some type of greater assistance, but did not know where to turn for help.

Family and friends offered their support, but Carolyn could not have stood the confusion of guests in the house. It would

47

have caused too much turmoil. It was hard to get her up in the morning and hard to get her going. Another person in the house was not the answer to this complex situation. Mary-Jane did not want Zachary passed from one person to another; she wanted him in as calm an environment as possible so he would feel safe. This was a big order in her current situation but a very important goal. One she was determined to carry out.

Mary-Jane was anxious for the baby to bond with Carolyn. He had been bonding with his dad every evening and Demian was certainly the doting father, feeding him, changing diapers and giving him his loving attention. In an effort to have him bond with Carolyn, Mary-Jane would wait until Carolyn was calm and then she got her together with Zachary. She said, "Then I would encourage her to interact with him and to sing to him while feeding him. This created a very positive interaction. It did not matter how short a time it was, it just needed to occur."

Mary-Jane's wisdom, tenacity, determination and her amazing stamina were important factors during these harrowing circumstances. She kept close to Carolyn, watching her every move, analyzing each change and desperately trying to move on to a solution. She found herself being the sole caregiver for Carolyn and Zachary, and sometimes Demian. At the same time, she felt as though she was making a superhuman effort, through sheer determination, to find an answer to what now seemed an insolvable problem. But Mary-Jane was not a person to give up easily; she had the same indomitable spirit her daughter had. Carolyn had obviously inherited it from her.

Demian said, "I deferred to Mary-Jane's experience a lot; especially during those first few months when it seemed like nothing worked for us. I trusted her implicitly. It would not have been smart, and in retrospect, potentially disastrous to have ignored the instincts of the woman that raised Carolyn. There was rarely any time to discuss the constantly changing situation because I was busy at work, and when I got home I immediately tried to help where I was needed. Now I needed ear surgery and was depressed about adding to the already overwhelming situation we were all in. We were both carrying a huge burden, but Mary-Jane carried the heaviest load."

Because of this burden, Mary-Jane was exhausted, lonely and scared and found herself in the middle of a situation

Mommies Cry Too

without any end in sight. She was not sure where to turn. Demian was trying to hold down his job, under extreme stress, and was facing major surgery. Mike, her husband and Carolyn's father, was at his job in Madison. Mary-Jane talked with him every night. He really was her "rock" and she relied on him heavily for support. He wanted to be there with her, but that wasn't possible. Without him, though, she felt alone and was starting to come apart bit by bit.

She knew she needed some kind of immediate help so she allowed her sister-in-law and brother-in-law to come for a visit. They had a close relationship with Carolyn and they would be able to stay with Zachary while Mary-Jane took Carolyn to the hospital for her surgery. Also, her brother-in-law was a cook and he could help with the meals.

Carolyn's aunt and uncle came and stayed a week, and during that time she had her surgery and was assured she did not have cancer. She seemed to perk up with this news and loved having her aunt and uncle there. Her uncle cooked all her favorite dishes and they had a pretty good week. Mary-Jane felt that things were looking brighter. Maybe the surgery had been part of the problem, perhaps it had been weighing on her mind. Following the surgery, her aunt and

50

uncle left, and Carolyn was quickly back on her feet.

Shortly after they left, Mary-Jane noticed it was a beautiful sunny day and she suggested to Carolyn they take Zachary for a walk. Their dog walked along with them and Mary-Jane was feeling a bit more confident. She asked Carolyn what she was thinking about since she seemed a little quiet. She said, "I was just thinking that it would be nice if a car came along and just hit me and killed me then I would not have to be bothered with anything." Mary-Jane was stunned and now *she* was getting panicky. She thought to herself, "Oh, my God, this is what she is thinking and I thought she was getting better. What am I going to do? This is not getting any better. We make some progress and then, boom, just like that, we are back where we started from."

Chapter 6

Electric Shock Treatments

Desperate measures are needed

In the middle of all this turmoil, Demian needed to have his surgery, so his parents, Lois and Jim, offered to take him to John Hopkins University Hospital. They left on a Tuesday and during that time Carolyn's condition went rapidly downhill. By the time Demian returned home from having his surgery on Friday, they were in a crisis mode. What a homecoming for him!

Mary-Jane had called the psychiatrist earlier in the week and he told her to increase the dose of Paxil, but that did not seem to offer any improvement. To Mary-Jane, Carolyn appeared to be in immediate danger. She had been in emotional pain for three months now and her suicidal feelings were very potent. She called the psychiatrist again and told him they were not getting anywhere with the depression and anxiety. "Carolyn continually talks of suicide by saying, 'I

52

Mommies Cry Too

just don't want to live like this anymore,' and recently told me of her plan to swallow a lot of her pills and die in her sleep," she told him.

By this time Mary-Jane had developed a strong basic trust in this particular psychiatrist. When he recommended ECT (electroconvulsive therapy) treatments because he felt the medication was not working, she listened. He told her, "This is really the only alternative when medication doesn't work and medication does not work for some people. The ECT treatments can be done right here in Richmond, at a local facility that performs them every day. They will be one hundred percent effective and accompanied with short-term memory loss for a brief period of time." He also, mentioned there was an excellent hospital in Baltimore for the treatment of PPD, but they would probably not be able to take her right away, so that was not going to be an alternative.

Mary-Jane knew they were nearing the end of the line but it was still unbelievable to her that something so incredibly drastic needed to occur. Desperate for more information and sick at heart, Mary-Jane and Mike decided to get another opinion before they could agree to the ECT treatments.

Mommies Cry Too

They needed to find another resource.

Mike always had his yearly physical at Mayo Clinic in Rochester, Minnesota, so he called some of his contacts there. He spoke with David Mrazek, M.D., Chair, Department of Psychiatry and Psychology. Mike asked Dr. Mrazek for his advice concerning Carolyn's PPD and specifically how he felt about her current doctor's recommendations for ECT treatments.

As Dr. Mrazek started to offer an explanation, Mike turned the phone over to Mary-Jane so she could explain Carolyn's PPD in detail and how they had reached this level of desperation. Dr. Mrazek suggested bringing her to Mayo Clinic, or, like their present psychiatrist had mentioned, take her to the Clinic in Baltimore because it was closer to them. But Mary-Jane told him, "I don't see how I would be able to manage getting her to either one of these facilities. Someone needs to care for the baby and it can't be Carolyn's husband because he's recovering from recent surgery; plus Carolyn has already been hospitalized twice and is now in a very deteriorated state.

"In fact," Mary-Jane told Dr. Mrazek, "I'm not sure I can

Mommies Cry Too

keep her alive for the weekend. I'm actually on a suicide watch. We are in a desperate situation. Our psychiatrist here has carefully explained to us that when medication doesn't work, ECT treatments are often recommended." She continued telling Dr. Mrazek, "He also described the procedure and the side effects to us. I told all this to Carolyn and managed to convince her that the ECT treatments would work. She promised to get herself through the weekend because she now sees the ECT treatments as her only hope."

Dr. Mrazek then expressed to Mary-Jane that he agreed with her psychiatrist's plan for ECT treatments. He said ECTs are very useful for individuals who either cannot take medication or are resistant to medication.

After Mary-Jane finished the hourlong conversation with Dr. Mrazek, she and Mike discussed the matter in great detail and struggled with the decision to go ahead with the ECT treatments. They finally came to the conclusion there were no other alternatives and they needed to do this so their daughter could survive. They reluctantly made the appointments, in the Richmond hospital, for the treatments to begin the following week.

Mommies Cry Too

Demian also reluctantly realized they had no other alternatives. They had already tried everything they could think of and nothing had really worked. He was, however, in his heart, against the ECT treatments. He was afraid of subjecting his wife to such a radical procedure, and didn't feel he was in the right state of mind to be able to make the decision. In the short time he had been home from the hospital he had researched every aspect of ECT treatments, but he couldn't put his finger on why he was against them. In his mind they were bad and scary. They had very frightening connotations. Even after all his research he did not want to do it; but did not feel emotionally strong enough to fight the decision. He said, "I was recovering from major surgery and was physically and mentally exhausted. I'm sure I wasn't thinking clearly at the time and it was probably not a good idea for me to be fighting something that Carolyn's parents felt was necessary."

He added, "I also knew my feelings against them were coming from fear, but I knew Mary-Jane and Mike well enough to know they had thought it through from every angle. This was a very difficult time for me and I went along with their decision but had tremendous reservations about it."

Demian emotionally added, "By this time, Mary-Jane and Mike had, in a sense, become my parents as well as Carolyn's. They had treated me like their son as soon as we were engaged. We had a strong bond between us and I trusted them implicitly. At this point, I felt I needed to defer to their wisdom. Despite how fearful I was, in the end I think it was the right decision."

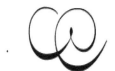

Chapter 7

ECTs were a Living Hell

They had reached the end of the line

The ECT treatments would consist of at least ten to twelve treatments, and involve the induction of an artificial seizure by passing a small amount of electricity through the brain for 30 to 60 seconds. Carolyn would be hospitalized for at least the first half of them and during the treatments she would not be uncomfortable because she would be under an anesthetic.

Carolyn leaves for her ECTs

Carolyn went to the hospital in Richmond for her first treatment on a Tuesday, and Mary-Jane went to see her on Wednesday morning. She was only allowed to have visitors once a day. Obviously, the short-term memory loss hit immediately because Carolyn kept saying, "Why am I here?" Mary-Jane tried to make her understand and explain-

Mommies Cry Too

ed to her over and over again why she was there, all to no avail. When Mary-Jane left to go back and care for Zachary, Carolyn called her every few minutes and begged to come home. On the Thursday morning visit it was more of the same, "Why am I here? What am I doing here? How do you know I have PPD, I don't remember that. I have not been depressed." Mary-Jane left again and Carolyn continued to call every five minutes saying, "Come and get me, right now."

Mary-Jane tried to get in touch with the nurse's station to stop her from calling, but she just got an answering machine. She later found out there was only one phone for the patients to use and it was located in the common room. Somehow, Carolyn was able to commandeer the phone by taking it out of the common room and then sneak into the kitchen to make the phone calls.

Mary-Jane relates, "In the midst of all this, I must admit to being briefly amused by Carolyn driving us all insane with her constant calling." She added, "When Carolyn was a teenager she loved the telephone. She would often be found lounging around the house talking to her friends on the phone. In fact, to this day she loves to talk on the phone, but

59

in this situation, the phone gave her comfort and was her link to her family. Somehow she had managed to bamboozle the hospital staff who had lost access to the phone because Carolyn was hiding with it and calling all her family and even her friends. Despite an extreme short-term memory loss she still managed to remember everyone's phone number. But, my amusement was short-lived due to the seriousness of her situation."

By the end of the week, Carolyn had quickly changed and had become very belligerent and demanding. It was horrible for Mary-Jane and there was nothing amusing about it. Carolyn would say, "You come and get me right now and if you don't, I am going to walk out and walk home." Mary-Jane said, "That was the most hellish day, the day I came closest to losing it myself." Mary-Jane was now in great despair and in tears most of the time. There would be no treatments on Friday, Saturday or Sunday.

The Saturday after Carolyn began the ECT treatments Mary-Jane's husband, Mike, and Carolyn's brother, Steven, arrived to assist Mary-Jane, who was now at her wit's end. Mary-Jane said, "Mike and Steven experienced similar agonies when visiting her. When they went in to see her she was

Mommies Cry Too

just horrible and very belligerent. She kept demanding to get out of the hospital. They tried to explain to her that each ECT builds on the previous one and the whole series, eight to twelve treatments, usually need to be completed, otherwise, the depression quickly returns. The explanation fell on deaf ears."

Her friend Jess had several phone conversations with Carolyn during her ECT treatments and said descriptively, "It was like the movie 'Groundhog Day,' where everything keeps repeating itself. Every time I talked with Carolyn she was confused, couldn't remember why she was there, and didn't remember being depressed. It was like someone continually pressed a reset button in her brain and wiped the slate clean of any information gathered in the hours before. She was basically like a caged animal, so completely desperate and scared that she would do anything to get what she wanted, including blackmailing her family. Even though her memory was being erased, she still knew her family well enough to know exactly which buttons to push to get them to crack. She was basically systematically breaking them down."

It was hard on all the family to visit Carolyn during this time but Demian bore the brunt of it. He had just been through a major operation and now he had to deal with visiting Carolyn on a daily basis and see the results of the ECT treatments. "I didn't like visiting Carolyn during the ECT treatments. It was just awful," he said with a heavy heart. "I did not actually see the treatments being done to Carolyn and that was a good thing, but I knew exactly what they were doing because of my research. Visiting her was like a nightmare, because when you're given an ECT treatment it sort of reboots your system and each time they gave one to Carolyn, she had no idea why she was there or what had happened to her. All this made her very frightened and scared. She was confused and at the same time she was angry at me because I wouldn't take her home. It was a very difficult position to be in and, frankly, it was very stressful for me. She pulled dirty tricks on me -- like I probably would have done -- to get me to take her home. She said things like, 'If you loved me you wouldn't leave me here. I can't believe you are doing this to me.' Her back was against the wall. It was absolute hell and I think the worst thing I ever had to deal with in my life and I had to go through this every day she was in the hospital."

After her fifth or sixth ECT treatment, Carolyn's difficult

Mommies Cry Too

and belligerent behavior continued and became a real problem for the hospital staff. Not only had she taken charge of the patient's phone but she was uncooperative, unruly, and kept demanding to be released immediately, often threatening to get out of the hospital and go home. The staff decided to move her to the acute side of the ward where they could keep a better eye on her.

Demian said, "When they moved Carolyn to the acute side of the ward things did not really change, she just had more restrictive visiting hours. What did change, though, was the hospital staff's attitude toward her. They did not see her as willing to stay in the hospital on a volunteer basis. Also, they saw her as a danger to herself, to other patients, and even to the hospital staff, who knew it was imperative for them to complete her ECT treatments. They were also concerned if she did go home she would not only be a threat to herself, since she was still suicidal, but could be a threat to her baby. The consequences of her behavior, due to the ECT treatments, had created yet another crisis for our family."

The hospital decides to commit Carolyn

When this type of situation occurs in a hospital treating

Mommies Cry Too

patients with a mental disorder, a standard procedure that the hospital can request, by a local court, is that the patient be committed for at least 90 days -- subject to a judge's approval. This was the situation Carolyn and her family were faced with and it was incredibly frightening.

The hospital did decide they needed to commit Carolyn for at least 90 days and scheduled a formal hearing with a judge. An attorney was assigned to represent her. Demian quickly began researching these types of hearings.

After doing so, they decided as a family that they could not accept commitment because this would go on her permanent record and would be available to anyone doing a background check on her. Her family would have a diminished role in her recovery process and the hospital would have total control over her care for as long as they felt necessary. This possibility created panic in Demian, Mary-Jane and Mike. The doctors and the hospital had not been making any discernable progress in helping Carolyn and the thought of having them in charge was terrifying. The family was currently looking for other medical resources to turn to for help and did not want to be limited to these doctors and this hospital. They believed if she were committed, the crisis would get worse -- and fast; but commitment seemed both possible and probable.

Demian researched all the legal issues he could find regarding commitment in preparation for the hearing and shared everything he found with Mike and Mary-Jane. Mike was a shrewd businessman with a knack for problem-solving and Mary-Jane's strength and common sense had been a great resource. They needed to put their heads together and come up with a plan.

The commitment hearing

Since family members were allowed to witness the proceedings and speak on behalf of the patient, Mike and Demian found themselves nervously waiting outside the psychiatric ward of the Richmond Hospital the morning of the hearing. They only had a few minutes to talk to Carolyn's lawyer before being led through the locked double-doors of the facility. Once they got inside the patient visiting room it was soon turned into a court room. The lawyer, along with Mike and Demian, tried to get Carolyn to understand the seriousness of the situation. She was exceedingly uncooperative and only wanted to go home and would not listen to them.

Mommies Cry Too

She did not seem to understand her current circumstances.

Mike said to her very sternly, "Carolyn, this is a big deal. If you keep arguing with them about leaving on your own they will keep you here for a long time and we can't do anything about it."

Shortly after the proceedings began, the judge attempted to engage Carolyn by asking if she was willing to stay in the hospital. To someone who knew her, Carolyn's facial expression and body language alone were proof enough they were in trouble.

Mike explained, "The real Carolyn would have been charming and very diplomatic in that kind of situation. Instead, she looked at the judge like she wanted to kill him. It wasn't so much how she answered the questions as it was her tone of voice. Every response, to the judge, was rude." Carolyn refused to stay and demanded to be let out immediately.

"It was really disheartening," Demian said. "We had to sit and watch her fate quickly slipping away into someone else's hands -- someone we didn't trust."

The judge then asked for the hospital's opinion on the matter. In order to maintain a certain degree of impartiality, a doctor who wasn't involved in Carolyn's treatment plan spoke on behalf of the hospital. He firmly stated that Carolyn should remain at the hospital.

At this point, the judge gave Mike and Demian a chance to speak. They knew it was not going well, but weren't ready to give up. Instead of arguing directly with the doctor's opinion their plan was to offer a compromise. They asked that Carolyn be allowed to come home after a few more ECT treatments and promised to bring her back for the remaining treatments on an outpatient basis. This was something Mike, Mary-Jane and Demian had previously discussed and was supported by the information Demian had gathered in his research prior to the hearing.

The doctor immediately challenged their request. "What makes you think you can provide the kind of care she needs?" he asked.

This was the opening Demian had been waiting for. "For starters," he said, "we have myself, her father, her brother, and her mother all available to help, which is a far better

Mommies Cry Too

staff-to-patient ratio than you have here. Furthermore, we have no faith in your ability to keep her safe and healthy and would rather care for her ourselves."

When the doctor offered no response, the judge asked Carolyn if she would agree to stay a few more days on a voluntary basis, and then be released for outpatient care.

The silence between the judge's question and Carolyn's answer was deafening. "I remember silently pleading, 'Please say yes, please say yes' over and over again in my head. When she actually said, 'yes' my heart started beating again," Mike said.

Demian said, "I remember feeling so relieved, not because we won, but because we dodged a bullet. I'm sure things would have turned out very differently if we had not been prepared."

Demian credits his father-in-law for his strength that morning. "Now that I have a child of my own, I clearly understand how feral you can feel when your child is threatened. It was amazing how strong Mike was able to be that morning."

The hearing was another example of Carolyn's family sticking together in a crisis and doing the impossible. They came close to losing control of her care and perhaps losing her.

As an out-patient, Carolyn has her last 4 ECTs

"Carolyn had eleven treatments in all and the last four were done on an outpatient basis," Demian said. "A treatment was done every other day so she had been in the hospital for at least two weeks. We didn't see any real improvement; in fact, on one of her last days in the hospital, something very strange happened. I arrived dreading the agonizing mix of Carolyn's tears, anger and confusion, but this time she was downright manic. Not only did she gleefully introduce me to several of the nurses and patients, but at one point she hopped onto my lap and started making out with me. I like being kissed as much a the next guy, but given the radical behavior change and the setting, it was pretty uncomfortable."

By the time she came home, after having seven ECT treatments, she was no longer belligerent and demanding but more compliant and cooperative. On Saturday and Sunday they all noticed that Carolyn's emotions had flatlined. She

Mommies Cry Too

would sit in the rocking chair with no emotion on her face at all, just staring into space. This was very frightening. They all feared they had lost her and had made a horrible, horrible mistake. Mary-Jane called the psychiatrist and frantically told him, "My God! We have lost her, she doesn't have any personality." He said, "At this point in the treatments this is normal, and you have to trust me she will get her personality back."

Her friend Jess called her during this time and said, "It was like talking to a five-year-old. After I hung up the phone, I ran to my husband and started crying. I felt like Carolyn was permanently damaged and that her old personality was gone. I was devastated."

Mary-Jane said, "I just couldn't believe it. She had no emotions, she would sit for the longest time and had no memory of the treatments at all. I really didn't think we would ever get her back. This was the very worse point in this whole experience. Our daughter appeared catatonic; it was hell. I was so frightened," Mary-Jane cried as she added, "Over the weekend she improved somewhat, but I felt like I was going through a nightmare that was never going to end.

70

Mommies Cry Too

"On Monday I took her back, on an outpatient basis, for her eighth ECT treatment. She did begin to show some slight signs of improvement and the doctor kept assuring me that she would be fine.

"Despite his reassurances, it was almost impossible to see how she would come back from this state. Mike and I were starting to wonder if, in fact, anything would ever be fine again."

Around this time Mary-Jane decided to have a serious talk with Demian. She said, "If Carolyn doesn't come out of this and if she doesn't come back to her old self, Mike and I would support you moving on and making a new life without her. You are too young to be saddled with a mentally ill wife. This isn't what we want for you. We will always love you, no matter what you decide but it is something perhaps you should think about."

Demian didn't need to think at all. He vehemently stated, "Carolyn has always stuck by me through everything and I am not going to desert her now. I don't intend to give up while I have a breath left in my body. I love her and I believe that we will pull through this, it might take some time, but I expect to be there when she comes back to me." This is an incredible example of his unconditional love for Carolyn and that he never gave up.

Chapter 8

Caregivers Exhausted

Mary-Jane and Demian are completely exhausted

Mike was beginning to see the impact all this was having on Mary-Jane and he felt strongly that when the treatments were over, she had to come home for a rest. Maybe she could come back to stay with Carolyn again, but she needed to get her equilibrium back. So, Mike and Steven told her, "We are not leaving until you've made reservations for your flight home." They took her out for ice cream and said, "You're burning yourself out and will soon be sick yourself, and then we will have two major problems on our hands." Mary-Jane agreed to go home.

Mary-Jane said, "If they hadn't made such a point about this, I probably would have stayed and that wouldn't have been the right decision. I knew I was right on the edge of falling apart. After this decision was made, I realized I would have to find a nanny because Carolyn would not be

Mommies Cry Too

able to do everything on her own." She told Mike and Steven, "I don't exactly trust her with Zachary. In her current state of mind, I'm not sure she will even be able to take care of herself, let alone remember to feed, change and tend to the baby."

"Guardian Angel" arrives

How was Mary-Jane going to find a wonderful, reliable nanny who could handle all these difficult problems? It seemed like an impossible task, but so far she had been doing the impossible and battling against the odds. This time the odds were with her. She opened the phone book to the Yellow Pages and under ads for "Day Care" she saw an advertisement that jumped out at her. It said "Postpartum Care." She called and was told they had just the person for her. This particular person was good with babies and was free to begin when they needed her. Mary-Jane asked her to come right over for an interview.

Mary-Jane said, "I knew the moment I saw Betty get out of her car and begin walking up to the house that this was going to work out. I just knew she was the right person for the job. These feelings only intensified when we began to talk." Mary-Jane had very good instincts about Betty, who

Mommies Cry Too

just radiated kindness and gentleness. Thankfully, her instincts proved to be more than accurate.

Mary-Jane poured out all her concerns about Zachary to her. She emphasized, "Zachary needs to be kept safe and calm and lately he hasn't been as interested in his bottle for some reason. It is an effort to get him to take his formula and you have to really be persistent. Do you think you can handle all this?" Betty said she thought she could. Mary-Jane decided to test her. She made an appointment to get her hair cut and left the baby in Betty's care. When Mary-Jane returned Betty was feeding Zachary, who seemed very calm and secure. Mary-Jane hired her immediately.

Mary-Jane then began to prepare Betty for Carolyn by elaborating on Carolyn's PPD. She explained, "The person you will be taking care of, besides Zachary, is my daughter, but she is not the daughter I've always known. She is just a different person. She's suffering from severe PPD and has significant memory loss from the ECT treatments she just had. The memory loss is so extensive she cannot be expected to do simple procedures for the baby, like feeding and diaper-changing because she doesn't remember how. It's hard for me to describe Carolyn since she has had most of her ECT

75

Mommies Cry Too

treatments, but she has become unreliable and can't be trusted to use her instincts like holding the baby with one hand while changing him, so he won't fall. Also, she seems to have no personality. It is very difficult to comprehend and has been difficult for me to watch."

Betty could see how hard all this had been for Mary-Jane. She felt sorry for Mary-Jane because she knew how tough it was going to be for her to leave Carolyn. But Betty knew, instinctively, it was the right time to put a fresh face on the current situation; she hoped Mary-Jane would realize this and that would help her face the prospect of leaving her daughter.

Betty asked Mary-Jane, "How did you ever get through this?" Mary-Jane said, "At first I didn't want to tell anyone, thinking that this situation wouldn't last very long, but then I soon realized I was in this for the long haul. My close friends called me often and offered support. Just talking to them helped. My husband, Mike, has been so supportive, I talk to him every day and he really has kept me going and tried to keep me positive. Also, Zachary is a very good baby and he didn't have a brother or sister that needed my care. He rarely fussed and slept through the night sooner than most babies. If he had been a difficult baby, I'm not sure I would have made it. Certainly, I would not have been able to handle it by myself."

Betty said, "I felt great sadness in my heart for Mary-Jane and her family." She added, "The complete despair in Mary-Jane's face was obvious and I knew I needed to try to help. She was completely exhausted and totally drained of energy. I felt it was my responsibility to add a new perspective to these circumstances."

Betty was very concerned, though, because she had no training for the extreme case of PPD that Mary-Jane was describing. In fact, Betty had taken care of many babies and mothers who were very stressed-out and tired but she had never been asked to take over anything quite this desperate. Betty told Mary-Jane she would really try to help but was worried about her ability to handle the situation because she had never taken care of anyone with PPD. Mary-Jane said, "It will be all right, just be yourself, you'll be fine." She added, "Carolyn doesn't need someone with special training, she only needs a companion, someone who will be there to help her and to make sure Zachary is getting the attention he needs. She has the instincts of a good mother,

Mommies Cry Too

they are there even in the depths of depression, they just need to be brought out."

Mary-Jane intuitively had confidence in Betty and her instincts proved to be correct. Betty would take over Mary-Jane's role, one that she could no longer do, but a role that was well-suited to Betty. It can't be overlooked, however, that Betty was a very brave person taking on this huge responsibility. When asked how she had the courage to do this, her response was, "Because I believe in hope, and I was very hopeful I could help turn this situation around."

Betty meets Carolyn for the first time

With some trepidation on Betty's part she finally met Carolyn for the first time. She said, "The one thing that really stood out for me were her eyes, they were so incredibly sad. I would later learn (when Carolyn was well) that you can learn everything you need to know about how Carolyn is feeling through her eyes -- happy, sad, angry, or whatever. But I didn't know that then and all I could think was how big and sad they were." She added, "At that early stage, our relationship was awkward and I didn't want her to feel that I had put myself in charge of her baby. She seemed to somewhat resent the need for my presence and I'm not sure she liked me very much. I knew she was afraid, nervous and scared. Her mother had described her as a strong-minded person, so I tried to imagine myself in her position. It would be difficult to admit I needed help and how was this stranger going to help me."

The primary focus of Betty's job was to take care of Zachary, to keep him safe, well-fed and on a daily schedule. Carolyn would routinely give Zachary his lunch, and then she would go upstairs and take a nap. She still had three more ECT treatments to take as an outpatient and Mary-Jane would stay until they were completed.

Carolyn's memory began to return toward the end of the ECT treatments. But when she looks back at this period of time, she barely has any memory of Betty being there.

Mary-Jane continued caring for Carolyn until the ECT treatments were completed. Every day, when Carolyn came home from her treatment, she would forget about Betty being there to take care of Zachary and every day, Mary-Jane would remind her why she was there. Betty took this all in stride, like there was nothing unusual about it.

Carolyn finished her ECT treatments on a Monday and Mary-Jane returned to her home on Wednesday. When she left, Carolyn was not catatonic anymore and seemed better and more aware of what was going on. Her mind seemed to be waking up a bit and her mother began to see some aspects of her old self returning. Carolyn continued to have problems with short-term memory loss but her personality was coming back. Mary-Jane felt better about her progress but realized she had not recovered one-hundred percent. She wasn't completely comfortable leaving at this point, but knew she had to go home for a while. Mary-Jane was physically and emotionally exhausted and knew she couldn't do any more until she had some rest.

It turned out that Betty was a wonderful nanny for Zachary, and was an integral part of Carolyn's recovery. Due to Betty's strong faith she believed that it was God's hand that brought her to this family so she could not only help this family, but also understand the serious damage this illness can cause to a woman and her loved ones. She became their "Guardian Angel."

Chapter 9

Appeared ECTs Failed

More bad news

Mary-Jane arrived home on a Wednesday. She was finally starting to feel somewhat rested when the unthinkable happened. They had been assured by both Carolyn's psychiatrist and Mayo Clinic that the ECT treatments would likely be highly effective. On Sunday night, however, Demian called and said they had a very bad weekend. Carolyn was talking about suicide again and she kept saying she couldn't handle the baby. He said, "She is not as bad as she has been," but he emphasized, "it appears to me the ECT treatments didn't work." Mary-Jane was stunned and all she could think of to say was, "That is just not possible. How can this be happening?"

Mary-Jane had been home for four days and they were in deep trouble again. She called the psychiatrist and asked him if this was normal. He told her it wasn't. She asked

Mommies Cry Too

him, "What do I do now? Should I send her to this clinic in Baltimore or Mayo Clinic?" He said, "I would encourage you to get another opinion." This doctor was obviously at the end of the line with treatments he could offer Carolyn and he really had no further recommendations.

At this point, Carolyn's family, and especially her father, Mike, were overwhelmed with frustration and absolutely desperate. Mike said, "After four months of no progress, I was discouraged and getting angry. There had been the failure of three different series of medications and the failure and horrible experience of the ECT treatments, plus the fact that the doctors who were taking care of her had basically given up. We were now facing a huge crisis because we did not know how to help her."

Finally, in desperation, Mike called Dr. Mrazek (who had talked with them about the ECT decision) at Mayo Clinic and told him, "No one has been able to help my daughter. We are at the breaking point here. What if we never get her back, what if she does something crazy? Why can't anyone help her? Why can't you help her?" Dr. Mrazek replied with conviction, "We will certainly do what we can to help her." At that moment, Mike sensed their luck was going to start to

Mommies Cry Too

change. The decision was made to get Carolyn admitted as soon as possible.

Mayo Clinic is their last hope

Mary-Jane expressed to Mike, "I guess that means I'll have to go to Carolyn's home in Richmond and take care of the baby when she goes to Mayo Clinic." Mike said, "No, you are staying here at our home and they are going to all come here. We'll deal with it here in Madison. At some point, we have to think about our own health and sanity. This has been going on for almost five months now." They settled in for an anxious wait for Carolyn, Demian and Zachary to arrive. Mike would then take Carolyn to Mayo Clinic, Mary-Jane would care for Zachary and Demian would have to go home by himself.

Betty keeps a close eye on Carolyn and Zachary

Before Carolyn left her home for Mayo Clinic, Betty kept close to her. Betty said, "I didn't know what to expect or what type of person she was, since I hadn't known her before. All I knew was what Mary-Jane had told me about her before PPD had set in. I knew she was really sick so I

83

Mommies Cry Too

was very cautious and watchful for her, as well as the baby. When Carolyn went up to her room to rest and closed the door, I was particularly concerned; so, I often went upstairs and stood by her bedroom door and listened to see if I could hear anything. I never did, so I assumed she was asleep, but I always gave a great sigh of relief when I heard her come out of her room."

Carolyn's friend, Jess, talked with her periodically during this time before she went to Mayo Clinic and gives us some perspective as to what Carolyn was thinking. It was absolutely frightening. She told Jess she had begun stashing her medication and was trying to save up enough so that she could kill herself. She had two concerns: She needed to take enough medication that would be sure to kill her, not just put her to sleep for a long time -- and she needed to plan when she could take the medication so there would be enough time for it to work before someone discovered her and took her to the hospital. But she also had to figure out how she could get all this done and not leave the baby unattended for too long, so that nothing would happen to him while this was going on. According to Jess, she was researching this on the Internet. Fortunately, Carolyn was not able to put all the pieces of this plan together but the possibility that she might

Mommies Cry Too

have is terrifying and indicates her continued severe depression and despair. Jess knew she was leaving for Mayo Clinic shortly and prayed she would make it there and that they could find a way to bring her back.

Betty, of course, did not know what was in Carolyn's mind or how desperate she actually was, but she was observing her very closely. She said, "After the ECT treatments, her personality was negated for a while and she just didn't have her wits about her; or I guess you could say she didn't have her complete mind back. At that time, she lacked the ability to care for the baby properly. She was really in pretty bad shape.

"Carolyn did, however, try to help with the baby and since Zachary sometimes fussed about taking his bottle she would often say, 'Let me try.' I could see she was trying hard to help but could clearly see her heart was just not in it. Zachary wasn't very interested in his bottle and that did not help the situation." Betty added, "I had never seen a baby that refused his bottle and I thought perhaps the feeding problem was a reaction to Carolyn's PPD or a part of it."

For Carolyn, Betty was the right person at the right time.

Mommies Cry Too

Betty did not realize how severe Carolyn's condition was, and perhaps because of that, she was able to surround her with a positive attitude and Carolyn needed that. It was helpful to have someone caring for her who had not been there during the earlier part of her PPD, and who was not anxiously looking over her shoulder every minute saying, "Are you O.K.?" and "What's going on with you today?" Betty was keeping an eye on her but was not judgmental. She always kept a low profile and was very kind and understanding. She never forced Carolyn to do anything, but would make suggestions regarding the care of Zachary and she would always compliment her on her mothering skills. She would make comments like, "I really liked the way you handled Zachary," or "You're a good mother." She built up Carolyn's confidence in a natural way and had also fallen in love with Zachary. That had made a huge impression on Carolyn.

The Saturday before she left for Mayo Clinic, Betty went to Carolyn's home and told her she would pray for her, that she had strong feelings of hope, and truly believed she would fully recover. Carolyn really needed all Betty's prayers and kind words of hope and encouragement. Fortunately, those prayers would be answered and Carolyn would find the hope at Mayo Clinic she was so desperate-

86

ly looking for.

When it was time to leave for Mayo Clinic, all three of them, Carolyn, Zachary and Demian, were to fly together on a plane to Mary-Jane and Mike's home in Madison. The day before the flight Demian had been sick in bed all day. He had developed "stomach migraines," which made his stomach cramp up and then he would be sick to his stomach. This, of course, was due to the incredible stress he was under. His hope was that if he stayed in bed the day before they left he would feel better for the flight. He knew it was his responsibility to get Carolyn and the baby to her parents' home. So, on the day they were to leave, he dragged himself out of bed and got Carolyn and the baby packed. "At the same time," he said, "I was noticing that Carolyn seemed anxious to get to Mayo Clinic because, I was beginning to sense, she wanted to get better. I felt somewhat encouraged. We all piled into the car and then I proceeded to throw up in the driveway, but somehow was able to pull myself together enough to drive us to the airport.

"When we arrived at the airport Carolyn realized I was in pretty bad shape, so she took over and managed to get us on the plane. We had a connecting flight in Atlanta and I felt so sick and completely out of it, but somehow Carolyn managed to get us on the right flight."

Carolyn was still able to focus on Zachary

Demian realized how incredible it was that Carolyn had pulled this off in her current condition. She was really still very sick, but she had dug deep and found the strength. He was so proud of her. He starting thinking about what she had been through and how she often managed to somehow pull it together for Zachary, albeit in small ways, but, huge in the end. Demian said, "The amazing thing about Carolyn, even when she was deep in her PPD, whatever energy she had left she would focus on Zachary. Even when 99.2 percent of her faculties were gone the .8 percent was directed toward him. If it was possible for Zachary to remember how his mom treated him when he was just a few weeks old and someone asked him, he would say, 'I didn't see her as much as I expected to, but every time I did she was smiling and laughing.'" Demian added, "Sometimes it may have been forced. But she made a tremendous effort to focus on him when she could, to keep him happy and make sure he was all right."

Demian continued, "Where she got the strength in the condition she was in, I don't know, but because of her incredible determination, she got us all to her parent's home in one piece. She was amazing."

Mike and Mary-Jane picked them up at the airport and took them to their home. Demian was still sick, so he went directly to bed. Mike left with Carolyn to drive her to Rochester, Minnesota, where Mayo Clinic is located, and Mary-Jane got busy caring for the baby. It seemed that this nightmare would never end. Zachary was more than four months old and the whole family was on the edge of an emotional collapse.

Chapter 10

Carolyn arrives at Mayo Clinic

Carolyn is admitted - diagnosed with major depression

When Mike called Dr. Mrazek and poured out his desperation, frustration, and anguish about Carolyn's experience with PPD he was very relieved to know Carolyn gained admittance at Mayo Clinic. There, she saw Dr. Mrazek and Grant Bauer, a Clinical Social Worker from the Department of Psychiatry and Psychology. Grant gathered the initial information for Carolyn's admittance and the clinical information from her former health care providers. He reviewed all the information and met with Dr. Renato D. Alarcon, Medical Director of Mayo Clinic Psychiatry and Psychology Treatment Center and its Mood Disorder Unit, who would be the treating psychiatrist on Carolyn's medical team. They both reviewed the information that had been gathered on Carolyn, and Grant said, "The medical team concurred that we had a pretty good idea, even before we met her, of what type of case we would be treating."

Carolyn had arrived at Mayo Clinic in a devastated condition and was cognitively impaired. Her memory was very poor and she was in a state of major depression, which can, in itself, cause memory and thinking problems; plus, she had recently received eleven ECT treatments, which can also cause significant memory problems. The Mayo Clinic medical team felt her previous diagnosis of PPD with borderline psychosis was a bit ambiguous, and did not see any overt signs of psychosis, dispite the obvious vulnerable state she was in. Instead, the team saw typical PPD symptoms, now enmeshed within a major depressive disorder diagnosis.

At Mayo Clinic's Mood Disorders Unit, PPD is treated as clinical depression because it presents the same symptoms. However, there are differences; the onset follows birth and sometimes, as in Carolyn's case, the onset followed Zachary's birth almost *immediately*. Also, there is an obvious hormonal component.

Dr. Alarcon stated, "On the day Carolyn was admitted, I interviewed Carolyn and her father. Her father told me that for at least a year and a half, including the time of the pregnancy, he noticed changes in Carolyn's behavior and demeanor indicating added tension, anxiety, and hypersensitivity -- that type of thing. She also had (pre-cancerous cells) on her cervix, and nothing could be done about that until after the baby was born." Dr. Alarcon continued, "Anxiety before birth can increase your sensitivity to clinical depression or PPD because it's closely connected in a time continuum; and life events can add to the severity of depression." Also, Carolyn's strong personality, as previously described by her father, was both a positive and negative component in this situation. In her case, though, Mayo Clinic felt that her personality features, being more positive than negative, would be prognostically favorable, and clearly contribute to saving her.

Given the severity of Carolyn's depression, she was facing several difficult issues at once. Among these were the side effects of the antidepressant medications, as well as the stress of parenting a newborn baby. At this point, she was unable to function in many of the ways she had so effortlessly been able to before. Her situation was severe.

Carolyn's medical team at Mayo Clinic would consist of five people whom she would see every day: Dr. Alarcon, the treating psychiatrist; Grant Bauer, the clinical social worker; a physician's assistant; a registered nurse; and a clinical nurse specialist. Occasionally, she would see an occupational therapist or recreational therapist. This team was indeed multifactorial, multidimensional, and multidisciplinary.

Did Carolyn meet the PPD clinical standard?

Carolyn met the clinical standard for PPD and there seemed to be no question about that. Dr. Alarcon said, "PPD is a very enigmatic condition with some contradictory findings. We know there are four dimensions: genetic, biochemical, hormonal, and personality-based or psychological traits." She seemed to have them all. She had a *genetic* predisposition to depression on both the maternal and paternal sides of her family and appeared to have some previous *hormonal* sensitivity to estrogen. There seemed to be some indication of anxiety two years prior to the birth which could cause *biochemical* malfunctions in the brain making her more susceptible to depression and she also had *strong personality traits*, and described herself as "type A".

What Carolyn was thinking when admitted

When Carolyn entered Mayo Clinic she thought her depres-

Mommies Cry Too

sion was caused by the birth, and that what she needed were the right pills to get everything back in balance. She said to herself, "They need to fix me and send me home." The first time she saw her psychiatrist, Dr. Alarcon, she told him, "Give me the right pills so I can go home and be all better." He was shocked at her comment and said, "Carolyn, this is a multifaceted problem. It does not just require pills but will also require extensive therapy. There is a reason that this happened to you and you may not know what it is yet, but you need to address all of it." She was just furious with him and let him know it, because she wanted to take some pills and go home. But there would be a lot of hard work ahead for Carolyn, and she needed to put her anger aside and turn her energy toward getting well again. Her desire to recover was very strong, so she reluctantly complied.

Adjusting to her surroundings wasn't going to be easy. Carolyn remembers realizing that she was in the psych ward and she was initially terrified. "I couldn't get my mind off that. This was the first time I was fully conscious of what was going on around me and it was incredibly surreal, totally embarrassing, frustrating, scary and every other emotion you can think of," she said. "I was thinking about the people who were behind the doors in my hall. Would they be totally crazy? Would they scare me? Would I be safe here?"

"For some reason, right at this low point, I thought of Demian and how much I loved him and how he made me feel safe. I remembered what he said when my energy was almost totally gone and when I was in the deepest depths of despair, I still gave everything I had left to be sure Zachary was all right. Remembering that gave me a lot of strength that day." But her depression and despair were still part of her and she was pinning all her hopes on Mayo Clinic to pull her out of it.

Carolyn reaches out to her friend Jess in great despair

During her first day at Mayo Clinic's Mood Disorders Unit, there was a very sad event demonstrating Carolyn's ever-present feelings of despair. Carolyn called her best friend, Jess, who lived in Minnesota and told her she wasn't sure she could continue being Zachary's mother. She said, "It's just too difficult for me. I need you to promise to take him for me and raise him." Jess could not believe what she was hearing and was talking to Carolyn through her tears. She tried in vain to get Carolyn to talk with Demian about this, but Carolyn said she wouldn't and got more and more angry.

She begged her to promise that she would take care of Zachary no matter what. Eventually Jess did promise but got off the phone crying and once again devastated.

What happened to Demian?

Demian said, "Shortly after we arrived at Carolyn's parents' home, her Dad and Carolyn drove to Rochester and her mother got very busy caring for Zachary. I was so sick I had to spend a few days in bed before I flew home. When I finally got home I think I slept for two days, then went to work, came home, and slept some more. I followed that routine for a few weeks. My fellow workers were very sympathetic and understanding. The time for rest was such a gift! We had all been through such an incredible ordeal, and so much of it was just an agonizing blur to me.

"I spoke with Carolyn every day and that was the best gift of all. It finally felt like someone knew what they were doing and I started to really think she was finally going to get better. The medical team put together at Mayo Clinic was very professional; they were in charge, and it seemed like they were beginning to put the pieces of our life back together. I felt like she was being expertly taken care of, and because I knew Carolyn so well, I knew she would be working hard along with her medical team to be healthy and strong once again.

"Carolyn would spend three weeks at Mayo Clinic and then three weeks at her parent's home before I saw her again. That seems like a long time, but I really needed to put myself back together and I was able to stay in close touch with Carolyn and monitor her recovery."

Finally, Carolyn's recovery begins

Carolyn's team at Mayo Clinic would begin the recovery process by first getting her medication under control. Then they started using congnitive behavior therapy to start rebuilding her mental processing. She would meet with her medical team every day, as well as her support group.

Chapter 11

Mayo Clinic ~ Medical Breakthrough

Major medical breakthrough helps Carolyn

Carolyn would become a beneficiary of a major medical breakthrough. A few months before she arrived at Mayo Clinic, a new test called cytochrome P450 had been cleared for clinical use. Dr. Mrazek, in partnership with Mayo Clinic's Department of Laboratory Medicine, worked with Dr. Dennis O'Kane and others to develop cytochrome P450. This test helps to pinpoint genetic factors that may affect a patient's response to various drugs including several antidepressant medications. It also represents a major advance in the ability to provide patients with the best possible care for depression.

The genetic test measures how well a person will metabolize drugs. For example, if a person's body metabolizes a drug too slowly, the drug will reach excessively high levels in the body, and cause unwanted side effects that may be toxic.

If a person metabolizes a drug too quickly, the drug may be eliminated from the body before therapeutic levels are reached. This test allows a physician to predict a person's response to antidepressant medications and to reduce or eliminate possible negative side effects caused by them. This methodology is included in the science of pharmacogenomics, which is the study of genetic profiles of individuals and the way they process or metabolize compounds including medications.

Cytochrome P450 helps Carolyn

Mayo Clinic did a full medical analysis of Carolyn to determine the overall condition of her health and to see if something might have been misdiagnosed.

One of the first things they did was administer the metabolic test cytochrome P450 to determine why medication was not working for Carolyn. By doing a a simple blood test they discovered that she is an intermediate to slow metabolizer, which makes her one of the few people who cannot handle antidepressant medication dispensed in the normal manner. Mayo Clinic, at the time she was a patient there, was the only facility in the world using this test.

Mommies Cry Too

From 2000 to 2003, Mayo Clinic, according to Dr. Mrazek, had been studying patients who were having difficult reactions to medications, to see if they could determine why. Prior research had been conducted on this subject, and with that information and what they compiled, the doctors began to come up with the answer. After only three years of research, Dr. Mrazek felt Mayo Clinic had sufficient evidence to begin using the cytochrome P450 test on a clinical basis. In April of 2004, Mayo Medical Laboratories began accepting specimens for testing. Carolyn was a patient there in September 2004.

Dr. Alarcon said, "If the slow metabolizer takes an average dose of antidepressant medication, that patient is going to develop significant side effects that may be very severe and very bothersome. That is what is meant by toxicity. These side effects can actually increase the severity of depression." Since Carolyn proved to be an intermediate to slow metabolizer, it meant that the dose of antidepressant medication she was taking, which was in the normal range, would eventually become toxic to her. This explained why some of the medications she took worked for her briefly and then stopped working. The doctors who had previously prescribed medications for her would typically start her at a low

Mommies Cry Too

dose and then raise it to a higher level. In her case, the higher dose would become toxic and make her PPD worse instead of better. For someone who was a normal metabolizer, the medication would, most likely, have worked.

Dr. Alarcon said, "This particular medical advance was significant in Carolyn's case, because she had gone through three different drugs, and each time that they raised the dose, her symptoms got worse and her condition deteriorated." Because Carolyn's test showed she was an intermediate to slow metabolizer, doctors gave her Effexor a medication she never had before. They started her on a low dose and then increased the dosage level, but kept it in the lower range. This really helped her."

Carolyn's case included a number of other factors in addition to medication, but the medication was definitely a major factor. She adjusted well to the dose, and did not need an increase. She also started taking a medication that offers good anti-anxiety effects, and responded well to that medication. This became part of her positive response to Mayo Clinic's treatment plan.

Carolyn and her family finally had an explanation why

Mommies Cry Too

nothing had worked for her. Their sense of relief, that she was finally on a medication she could tolerate and that would help her, was profound. They are convinced the test, cytochrome P450, helped save her life.

Dr. Mrazek elaborated further on the test: "Mayo Clinic continues to do a lot of interpretation on the test data. The interpretation can seem simple on one level, and complicated on another because metabolism is on a continuum. One can have no activity, slow activity, normal activity, somewhat enhanced activity or super-enhanced activity. So learning about the specificity of an individual's level of metabolic ability and the different drugs available to that individual is a learning process. Since we now have several years of experience with this test, we often provide consultation to other physicians at different treating facilities. When they get the results, and learn that their patient is an intermediate to slow metabolizer, we can then advise which drug would give their patient the maximum benefit."

Cytochrome P450 is now widely available

The manufacturer of the equipment for the test obtained FDA approval in the summer of 2005. This was the first time the FDA approved a genetic assessment device related to medication. Mayo Medical Labs worked with the manufacturer on an interpretive system to help psychiatrists interpret the results of the cytochrome P450 test.

The test is now widely available and is being used in the U.S., Europe, and the Netherlands.

Chapter 12

Cognitive Behavior Therapy

CBT is a major leap in Carolyn's recovery

Cognitive behavior therapy (CBT) was a major part of Carolyn's recovery in addition to correct medication levels, Grant said. "CBT is a form of psychotherapy based on the idea that feelings and behavior result from how one thinks about oneself and one's life. It focuses on recognizing negative thoughts or inaccurate beliefs a person may have about himself, a situation and their ability to cope. It helps challenge and replace those thoughts and beliefs with more positive and realistic ones so healthier attitudes, behaviors and habits can be developed," Grant explained. So, toward the end of her first day at Mayo Clinic, Carolyn got started on her CBT. She was, initially, a bit resistant but soon got enthusiastic about it because it started to make sense to her.

In an effort to get her negative thoughts out, Carolyn learned to write down her feelings. She remembers having an epiphany near the end of her first day at Mayo Clinic. She said, "I began by doing thought records on all the things I was afraid of. It turned out my negative feelings in every single record came down to the following thought: 'I am a bad mother.' I must have done eight or ten of these exercises where you write down a negative thought then you write under it what the thought really means. If you keep this process going usually you will discover what your subconscious mind is telling you."

Carolyn said, "In my waking mind, I didn't think I was a bad mother, but strangely enough my subconscious was playing a trick on me. It was a thought that was driving everything I was doing. My mind kept repeating to me, 'I am not a good mother, I am not a good mother.' It was like being caught up in a vicious mind-numbing circle, and I couldn't find my way out. For example, taking Zachary to the grocery store made me very nervous; consequently, I didn't want to take him. The resulting thought process was: I don't want to take him so I must be a bad mother, because everyone else is happy about doing it and thinks it's fun to take their child to the grocery store, but since I don't want to, so I must be a bad mother. That was the culminating negative thought."

Mommies Cry Too

She added, "That was my first day at Mayo Clinic, and I was given these exercises to do. Because I am normally very diligent about this type of thing, I took my unfinished work to my room to do as homework and finished all the exercises that evening."

The following day when Carolyn went to her support group with other depressed patients for the first time, she told the patients and therapist, "I have done my thought logs and I have concluded that I am a bad mother." The therapist challenged her by asking, "What proof do you have of that?" In Carolyn's case there was none because she was a new parent, and she hadn't even spent time alone with her child. The therapist asked her to challenge those thoughts and feelings with her family.

Carolyn said, "I remember calling Demian and my mother and telling them that I thought I was a bad mother." But then she quickly added, "Except I really think that is untrue -- I'm actually a pretty good mother." Her family, of course, reinforced that she was *not* a bad mother and felt she would make a wonderful mother. Carolyn knew in her heart she had tried her best, even in her deepest despair, to do whatever she was capable of doing for Zachary.

At last some <u>hope</u> dawns!

"From that moment, when I said, 'I am not going to accept that I am a bad mother,' because that was just not me, everything was different. I also knew I was in a safe environment at Mayo Clinic. I was being well-taken care of and in capable hands. It was clear to me my medical team knew what they were doing, and I started to develop confidence in them. It was really the first time that anyone was really in charge of the entire process. It was an enormous feeling of relief that I was finally with professionals who were going to examine me from every angle, and who would finally be able to help. I was getting a good feeling that this could be the turning point for me."

Demian remembered her phone call and said, "When Carolyn went to Mayo Clinic I began to have some hope because I had grown up in Minnesota and I knew of their incredible reputation. To hear her say, 'I knew in my heart that I was a good mom' and to say that on the second day she was there, well, I nearly cried. I finally had hope, too, and it has been uphill ever since. It was huge! This was the beginning of her recovery."

CBT is critical to Carolyn's recovery

Grant was able to explain Carolyn's epiphany by saying, "People with strong personalities often have trouble letting go of their negative thoughts. However, Carolyn was very studious and worked very hard on the methods the medical team gave her. It speaks well of her, because she did the lion's share of the work in examining her feelings and behaviors. She really used all the tools we made available to her to help herself out of this awful situation, for herself, her baby, her husband, and her family, and the providers on the multidisciplinary team."

Carolyn had a very tough depression. She didn't have a good result from many different medications, and she did not seem to respond well to the ECT. Her problem was certainly multifactorial. Finding out that Carolyn was an intermediate to slow metabolizer and getting her on the right medication was critical, but the CBT was equally beneficial for her in examining her character and her thought process.

"Each day I would meet with Carolyn, individually, in the latter part of the day so I could process with her how the group therapy went and what Dr. Alarcon was proposing.

Mommies Cry Too

She seemed to need that closing of the loop every day," Grant said.

Through her experience in group therapy it became clear to Carolyn how lucky she was to have such a supportive network of family and friends. Many in the group did not have, at their immediate disposal as she did, the resources for their recovery. She really began to count her blessings.

Having a 'type A' personality with some facets of being more on the obsessive side, meant that Carolyn may not have been prepared for a motherhood that was not going to go like clockwork. Zachary's rejection of the breast, for a person like Carolyn who wanted to do everything right, turned into a disaster. Then all the treatments that she reacted negatively to exacerbated the problem. Add to that a family history of depression and her cognitive decline, whether from the ECT or the depression, making her thought process and her memory impaired. Anyone who is faced with that situation is going to struggle. In her case, she had a very sharp mind and a clear sense of processing, along with being very intelligent and analytical. When these qualities were decreased because of her impairment, she *really* got anxious. "I am just not me anymore," Carolyn described.

109

Mommies Cry Too

Dr. Alarcon reiterated what Carolyn's father had said. "She has a stunning personality, always very sociable and energetic -- better known as a 'type A' personality." This is a healthy personality, a little on the extreme side, but not pathological. "In the medical literature we call this protective factors versus risk factors. This means the personality traits were ultimately going to protect the patient from the severity of the diagnosis, they were going to keep the diagnosis from happening, or they would help the patient recover better. Strong personality traits, like indomitable will, perfectionism, and self-confidence, are protective." These traits were positives, in the sense that Carolyn recovered because of them, and helped Mayo Clinic to predict a positive outcome. Instead of, for example, a woman who is lacking in self-confidence and has a dependent personality; this would make her more vulnerable, with possibly a less than positive outcome.

"Personality traits work like a double-edge sword because they also can contribute to the complications of PPD," Grant said. Carolyn was almost obsessive-compulsive about doing everything right. She was a perfectionist and wanted to be the perfect mother, and if she could not be perfect she thought she must be a bad mother.

"I did not agree with the former diagnosis that Carolyn had PPD with borderline psychosis," Dr. Alarcon said. "She had a very significant PPD. The symptoms she had indicated a typical PPD including a real fear of not being a good mother. Because she felt she was not a good mother, she did not want the baby nearby -- not because she rejected the baby but because she didn't believe she was a good mother.

"A psychotic mother, on the other hand, loses touch with reality and hates the baby, rejects him or her, and sees the baby as evil.

"Carolyn did not lose touch with reality but was terrified she couldn't be a good mother. Her recovery was really quite extraordinary. She had many things going for her, mainly her personality. In my daily contacts with her, I emphasized her strengths and tried to help motivate her and give her hope. Because hope is what is really going to get the patient back on their feet and moving toward recovery. The multi-dimensional view we have at Mayo Clinic is not just medication and therapy."

Treatment includes hope

Hope it appeared, became a powerful factor in Carolyn's

multidimensional recovery. Dr. Alarcon often referred to Dr. Jerome Frank's book, *Persuasion & Healing* because he was a student of Dr. Frank's at Johns Hopkins University. He emphasized, "Dr. Frank believed hope was an essential ingredient in healing." He says in his book, "The mobilization of hope plays an important part in many forms of healing, causing favorable expectations to generate healing; especially for those illnesses that have a large psychological or emotional component."

Chapter 13

Did the ECTs work?

ECTs remove the cloud over your mind

Carolyn wanted to know if the ECT treatments worked for her. She learned at Mayo Clinic that PPD is like a cloud or wall that comes down over your mind. The treatments break down that barrier and allow the chemicals in your brain to start working. The ECT treatments did work for her, but the problem was, since she was still taking antidepressant medication during the treatments, any positive effect they had was negated by the toxic levels of medication in her body. She could not effectively metabolize or eliminate the medication at the dosage level she was taking. This created a counter-productive situation; therefore, it was impossible to detect the positive benefits of the ECT treatments.

Carolyn was fascinated and encouraged by this explanation because she knew that after the ECT treatments some of her mental awareness did return, and her mind seemed to work

Mommies Cry Too

again. She also could remember now back to the last few ECT treatments. She was relieved she had them before she got to Mayo Clinic, because her mind was clearer, her long-term memory was returning, and that would obviously help her get better. Recovery was possible because there would be no more toxic levels of medication in her bloodstream, and the medication and dose level Mayo Clinic had pre-scribed would now have a real chance of doing its job. She once again sensed there might be some hope, as Betty had said when Carolyn left home.

Dr. Alarcon gives some history on ECTs

When Dr. Alarcon was asked about the ECT treatments, he stated, "The truth of the matter is that ECT treatments still, to this day, remain a mystery in what they actually do.

"When the ECT was used for the first time, more than 70 years ago, the explanations were non-existent, it just simply worked. One of the interesting observations at that time was that depression was not as frequent among epileptic patients as the normal population. So one astute scientist thought, 'If patients who have epilepsy don't have as much depression as the known population, perhaps the seizures that they have

Mommies Cry Too

are doing something to prevent it.' The clinical observation was, perhaps seizures would prevent or improve depression. So what is a seizure? Par excellance, it's an electrical charge. Which is exactly what the patient receives during an ECT treatment.

"Ultimately, it was found to be true that ECT treatments for most people would actually prevent or improve depression and they are used extensively today for just that reason."

Dr. Alarcon added, "With today's advances in biochemistry of the brain, including interaction of neurotransmitters and receptors, along with extensive knowledge of metabolism, genetics, and enzymes, there's a better understanding of the biological basis of depression -- by extension also the biological basis of PPD.

"Today we know that depression is related to a depletion or reduction of some of the neurotransmitters in the brain. Therefore, it's reasonable to assume that the ECT stimulates the production of neurotransmitters which are reduced, diminished or depleted in the brain or the central nervous system."

In depression, the ECT gives the patient a gigantic rearrangement in the biochemistry and functionality of the brain and it often results in less depression or a return to normality, Dr. Alcaron explained. Aftereffects, such as memory loss, can be very significant, but go away for the most part. "Today it's a very safe procedure." In Carolyn's case she received eleven treatments, which is close to the highest number -- twelve treatments -- given in one treatment period. "At Mayo Clinic, we monitor the treatments very closely and re-evaluate them on a continuing basis. If the memory impairment becomes significant, we stop, because the confusion and devastation that can result can be more disruptive than the depression," he said.

Carolyn's memory problems were significant and she was anguished by that. The change in her medication, and the change to a dose that was correct for her was crucial, but just as crucial was the CBT. That helped to speed up the recovery process, to rebuild her cognitive apparatus, and helped her biochemistry as well as her strong personality.

Carolyn was an acute observer of everything, so she was able to absorb a lot of information and learn quickly. Along with that she got a lot of support from her daily interactions

Mommies Cry Too

with all of us on her treatment team, and from other patients in the support group. "This kind of encouragement enhanced another very powerful element in her therapy, and that was hope. We all helped to rebuild hope in her, and hope begets motivation, and that was the best thing; her motivation to get better became very strong and that was another very important ingredient in her recovery," Dr. Alarcon added.

When Carolyn came to Mayo Clinic, she was devastated because of the depression and the postpartum remnants, disappointed about the ECT results, and disappointed about not being the mother she wanted to be, Dr. Alarcon said. "So, it was a gradual rebuilding and it was a positive result because of her positive personality factors and her good background," he added. "We needed to stimulate all this and bring it out, and we were very pleased with the result because she got what she wanted to be -- a good mother and to enjoy her baby."

Dr. Alarcon added, visibly moved, "After she left, she sent me a beautiful card, eloquently written, thanking us for giving her back her life and giving her back to her family and her child. Her recovery was an enormously powerful event.

She is a wonderful, strong person and she will be fine."

Carolyn spent three weeks at Mayo Clinic and another three weeks with her parents in Madison before returning to her own home. Mayo Clinic told her it could take up to a year to fully recover and feel like herself again.

Finally, Carolyn and her family had reason to be very hopeful. Recovery was fully under way. She was showing signs of tremendous improvement. Carolyn said, "It was the first time I felt really confident that I was going to get better. I knew the stars were aligning for me. I was on the right medication. I was starting to conquer my demons about being a mother. I was starting to care about life again (and the people in it). I just needed to keep the positive momentum moving forward and I could learn how to handle the rest. I knew I had a great support system and that gave me a leg up on most people. I felt stirrings of my old personality inside again and if I could just keep staying in touch with that, my old fighting spirit would guide the way."

Chapter 14

Carolyn gets her Life Back

Carolyn went home to complete her recovery

Carolyn was excited to be back home. Betty was back on duty to help her and said, "Carolyn became much more involved with the baby and I, of course, let her do whatever she felt she could. I tried not to interfere with her and Zachary after she returned home. She actually did most of the child care herself and I stepped in if she needed a short rest in the afternoons. Mayo Clinic had told her to try and rest every day as long as she felt she needed to. There was certainly a noticeable improvement in Carolyn and it was a pleasure to see."

Demian faces his fears

Demian was so excited to have Carolyn and Zachary back home and everything was looking so much better; but he was surprised to discover he was carrying some baggage and he knew was going to have to work hard to put things in their proper perspective. He had built up fears due to all they had been through. He also knew Carolyn better than Betty so he could see through her a bit. He said, "Carolyn seemed to be acting a little better than she really was, and I could see that. Sometimes I thought things were rather forced because she was trying so hard, but that was all right; she had lost so much time with the baby and was anxious to get everything back to normal as soon as possible. But, sometimes fear would grab me and I would think perhaps I was imagining that things were going better than they really were. We had been through so much, I couldn't help but think that maybe this was not going to work this time, either. So, I was dealing with some unexpected emotions that I had to wrestle with and resolve.

"I couldn't help looking back," he admitted. "I felt a lot of sadness, a lot of regret, probably some repressed anger and of course, I wished it never happened. I feared it would happen again and that I had to be ever-vigilant. I was afraid that something would trigger the PPD to return. Of course, that wasn't rational, but it was somewhat realistic, considering what we had dealt with."

He continued, "But some very good things had come out of all this. Zachary is just the coolest kid I have ever seen in my life. He is such a great little guy and doesn't seem scarred from all of the difficult turmoil he went through. It also brought to the surface that Carolyn needed to work on how she wanted to live her life, and resolved some issues for her, and helped her to move forward. It has helped her to become the person she wants to be. Not all bad. Personally, I feel if we could handle this, we can handle anything."

Demian said he began to work on his tendency to be hyper-vigilant because sometimes it was driving a bit of a wedge between Carolyn and him. "It didn't allow me the ability to relax and, consequently, didn't allow Carolyn to become a complete partner with me. This created tension. I knew it would go away in time, but I was holding on to it longer than I should have. The hyper-vigilance mixed with the normal frustrations of married life didn't make a good combination," he said. One of their frustrations was the fact that this was really the first time Carolyn and Demian had been alone as parents. They had to find their rhythm, like all new parents do, but they were doing it with a five-month-old, rather than a newborn. Fortunately, Demian was introspective and very observant. He recognized his fears and knew they were certainly understandable considering what he had experienced with PPD.

Demian continued, "I was always thinking, 'Is everything all right?' and would check up on her occasionally. If I couldn't reach her I would get worried. I wanted to know where she was practically all the time. When she was with her mom I knew she was fine, but when I knew she was home alone my mind would sometimes race with possibilities. I would imagine the worst and become very fearful. This caused me some very anxious moments, but I knew I needed to get beyond it and that would be critical to our total recovery. It was really post-traumatic stress to some degree, but perhaps not quite so vivid. But for the most part, considering where we were coming from and what we had been through, everything was going quite well. It was fantastic. Every day we saw progress.

"We were so fortunate to have Betty with us who was devoid of the baggage I was carrying. She was able to be much more positive than I was and really kept us all in the present. A present that was offering improvement every day, in large doses, and she helped us all to see beyond the rain and into the sunshine. Everyone needs a Betty! She truly was our "Guardian Angel".

Betty sees daily positive improvement

Betty said, "When Carolyn came back from Mayo Clinic she was at least halfway back to normal. She wasn't as sad and her confidence came back little by little. The sparkle returned to her eyes and I felt like I was a witness to a dramatic transformation as the weeks passed. Every day I could see more and more improvement in her." They started to do a lot of activities together and as Carolyn became more aware and more awake, a strong relationship developed between the two women. Betty became a surrogate mother to Carolyn and Zachary.

"There was a growing bond between Betty and I," Carolyn said. "One day Betty invited me to her house to make bread, because she thought it would be good therapy for me, but I thought it was more than that. I got to meet her husband and to know her in her own surroundings. The bread-making was fun but to me it signaled the beginning of a deeper friendship. She began to let me into her life and, of course, I just burrowed right in. She hasn't been able to get rid of me since."

Mommies Cry Too

Sometimes Betty had trouble adjusting to how well Carolyn had recovered. She said, "One day Carolyn said to me, 'I'm going to my doctor's appointment and Zachary's going with me, and on my way back I am going to stop at the drug store.'" Betty said, "I became very frightened, because it was a hot day and I was afraid she would forget the baby was in the car. Of course, this fear was a flashback to how Carolyn behaved after her ECT treatments when she had substantial memory loss. So, I guess you could say I over-reacted, and I had a little baggage of my own to deal with. Anyway she came back and they were both fine and I was very glad to see her." Betty added, "I realized this was a good sign and that her recovery was progressing well."

Carolyn finally overcome the fear of giving Zachary his bath; in fact, she gave him his bath before Betty arrived each morning. She also asked Betty many questions about the time they spent together after the ECT treatments and before she left for Mayo Clinic. Her memory of that time was rather hazy. To Betty, these questions indicated the former inquisitive Carolyn was back and she was getting to know the real Carolyn, the one her mother referenced long before when she said, "The Carolyn you are taking care of isn't my daughter." And Betty was beginning to love her very much.

Carolyn asked Betty a lot of questions about herself, about who she was and what her life was like. Betty said, "I could just feel her old curiosity returning. It did take awhile before I saw the bonding between Zachary and Carolyn begin; but, I watched it happen, slowly but surely, and saw the joy in Carolyn's eyes for her baby whom she really had not known before. She had no memory of him. It was incredible to see and a real spiritual gift to me!"

Carolyn said passionately, "Betty was so kind to me. It did not matter that I was almost 30 and she was 60, she was a Baptist and I didn't know what I was, but we had the same fun-filled spirit. We often had very serious conversations, but spent most of our time sharing laughter and happy times together. Betty was just nice and comfortable to be around and we really just enjoyed each other's company."

"One of the activities that Carolyn had a real problem with was shopping with the baby," Betty said. "It caused her great anxiety. She would do it, but it was so uncomfortable for her."

Carolyn knew Betty was aware of this anxiety, so when they did go shopping, Betty would make it seem like fun and not a big deal. She managed to remove the fear and replaced it with a relaxed, happy time. Carolyn said, "So I ended up not thinking it was scary to go to the grocery store with Zachary because Betty was with me and we just had fun. Soon the panic was gone and the scariness was forgotten. Then, all of a sudden, I was able to hop in the car, scurry off to Target or the grocery store with the baby and not need Betty with me. That was when I realized I was keeping her there for my company -- not because I needed her help anymore."

Normalcy returns - Betty leaves

Carolyn returned home from Mayo Clinic in October and by Thanksgiving she was a totally changed person. She helped prepare the Thanksgiving dinner at her home, and began to realize she had finally gotten her life back. Betty stayed with her and Zachary until the end of December. Since then, she has been a frequent visitor and will always be a dear and treasured friend. Carolyn feels that she, as well as Zachary, bonded with Betty.

Betty concluded, "Of all the people I have cared for, I never knew anyone who needed me more than Carolyn did. This need slowly turned to love, and I know that Carolyn and I will always have a special relationship. I also feel a special bond with Zachary, who is just a beautiful child and, truth be told, I fell in love with him the minute I saw him.

"I got to see Carolyn transform into a healthy, wonderful mother. It was miraculous, considering what she had been through. It was the happiest day of my life when she came to my house and said she didn't need me anymore. Carolyn cried and said she thought I was going to be sad, but I was joyful, and we had a wonderful celebration together.

"The last day I was there I told Carolyn she needed to go upstairs and take a nap. Carolyn said, 'This is the last day you will be here and I am not going to sleep through it.' So we got out the Trivial Pursuit game and played while Zachary slept."

Carolyn stated, "Betty left and I was comfortable and able to be a good mother, just like I always wanted to be. I knew some difficult days would lie ahead but I felt much more able to cope and my mind was working again. I started to think how some people are not lucky enough to even have one mother they love, respect, and cherish. But here I was, blessed to have the incredible mother that I have, who was my best friend and loved me so much that she gave up her life for six months to take care of my baby, and essentially saved my life and family. But, then I was lucky enough to have another amazing woman walk into my life and love me like a second mother. This woman too, would do anything for me, not to mention, Zachary and Demian. I sometimes can't believe my good fortune."

Chapter 15

They finally become a Family

Carolyn, Demian and Zachary are on their own

"After Thanksgiving," Demian said, "I remember feeling much more confident in Carolyn, but in December, we got off track for a while. Another serious operation was scheduled for my ear, and my parents came for a visit to help out and despite all they did for us, it was a little stressful having houseguests." After they left, Demian was still in recovery and Betty was preparing to leave. They had some chaos for a short time because Demian wasn't feeling well and it was an emotional experience for both of them to have Betty leave. She had meant so much to them during this difficult period in their lives. He said, "I knew we would go through an adjustment period and that made me a bit apprehensive. But by January we were back on track, on our own, and it felt good. I was feeling well, and less hyper-vigilant and I felt more secure in Carolyn's recovery; consequently, the first two months of the year were blissfully non-eventful."

Carolyn needs to forgive herself

It was fortunate that after Carolyn had left Mayo Clinic she found a local psychiatrist and psychologist to treat her during her recovery at home. Mayo Clinic wanted her to continue medication for at least another year so she needed the psychiatrist to prescribe this medication. She also needed to talk to a therapist once a week to keep track of her progress and to help her through some of the rough spots. She continued this therapy for about ten months, and during this time she was able to reduce her medication. Her therapist became crucial to her around March, when she let down her guard and admitted to Demian what he already knew, that she had been pushing herself hard to be better than she really was.

She confided to Demian, "My attitude, when I came home from Mayo Clinic had been to push all the bad stuff to the back of my mind, and move forward. I said to myself, 'I'm not going to cause the people I love any more problems.' Even though I had lost my memory from Zachary's birth to about three months later, it was not very hard to imagine the stress that I had caused everyone. So, I decided I was going to be better and I forced myself to be better. It was such a discouraging realization that this whole experience had taken so much time from my life."

Carolyn added, "It soon became clear to me that I had not given myself the time needed to mourn the loss of three months of memory, which included the birth of my son and the wonderful moments of his first few months of life. I had to listen to the story of my memory loss from my mom, my husband and Betty. Then, I needed to read about it in this book. Parts of the book I read along with my therapist in an effort to better absorb all that happened to me. That was pretty difficult, but something that was necessary for me to face."

Demian sadly added, "Periodically, she would emotionally break down a bit from trying to be up and happy and perfect all the time. Intermittently, she would get very upset that she had caused the most important people in her life so much stress -- the people whom she loved so dearly -- and that would make her feel very sad."

Carolyn describes her feelings at this time, "Whenever I had any fears, insecurities, normal mother feelings of fatigue, being overwhelmed, or sometimes even feeling a loss of

Mommies Cry Too

self, I would ignore those feelings, bottle them up, and then push them down and away. Since I am an incredibly emotional person at heart, this could only work for so long. Periodically, I would break down. Since I was storing it all up, it would be pretty significant. It would make the people around me very nervous. It became a problem, because the very thing I was trying to avoid (having the people around me worry about me) was exactly what was happening."

Carolyn said she needed to continue down the road to normalcy, and part of that was realizing that mothering is a very tough job. It's full of all sorts of complex feelings and emotions that don't have anything to do with PPD, but something that all mothers go through. She needed to get away from the baby for a couple of hours periodically. She needed more sleep and wanted to talk about adult things that weren't part of PPD. That was part of being a mom.

"My life had changed, but I hadn't. I still needed other people, a social life, and time with my husband. That was all quite normal. Once I started to admit it, schedule time away, talk about how I was feeling, I not only realized that other mothers (and Demian) felt exactly the same as I did because they wanted to get out and be themselves, too! After a while,

132

I didn't have breakdowns anymore. It was gradual, but it worked. It was about a year after I left Mayo Clinic when I finally felt like myself again," Carolyn said.

As Demian pointed out, " All this was very understandable. With Carolyn's mind totally back, this was some very hard stuff to deal with. She, of course, did not have PPD on purpose. Mary-Jane and Mike had moved on with their lives, and we needed to deal with this leftover trauma by ourselves.

"Once she came to grips with what she was doing, by trying too hard to be better than she really was, she started to see everything a little clearer and it explained why she was so emotional. It was important to understand that she could not just jump over all the misery that she and her family had been through, but she had to work her way through it. She had to face the guilt, forgive herself, and realize it was not her fault, and that is exactly what she did. Her therapist helped her through this period and she started to put the whole situation into a better perspective. Then she was able to move past it. That was the last chapter -- the end of the nightmare."

Mommies Cry Too

Tribute to Mary-Jane

Demian added, "This story cannot end without a tribute to my mother-in-law. We would not have gotten through this, we would not be sitting here today, if it had not been for her. Carolyn could have been dead, or institutionalized and we could have been divorced. Thank God Mary-Jane made the decisions she did. She was very decisive, and I trusted her. She had amazing fortitude and strength and kept moving toward the solution. She never once faltered, but was driven by her indomitable will to save her daughter and to get to the right answer. We were facing a huge multifaceted problem but somehow she kept moving us in the right direction. She is an amazing person and Carolyn and I are incredibly lucky to have her in our lives."

Gratitude to Mayo Clinic

Demian continued, "I don't know what we would have done without Mayo Clinic. They managed to put Carolyn back together, which in turn, put the rest of the family back together. I don't even want to think where we would be without them. We were very fortunate, and are very thankful to them."

Carolyn has the last word

"Whenever friends or acquaintances find out for the first time what I went through with PPD, their first reaction is to say, 'Carolyn, oh my goodness, what a terrible thing to have gone through. I'm so sorry that happened to you and your family!' Although I appreciate their kind words and sympathy, the funny thing is, I don't agree with them. Well, maybe on the surface, I guess it was a terrible thing to have gone through. But since I don't remember it, it actually was a lot worse for the people around me than it was for me personally. The thing is, I'm not sorry at all that it happened. That may sound crazy, but I'm actually thankful for what happened to me. Why? The reasons are so numerous that it is hard to know where to begin, but I can certainly list a couple.

"First, I am now so grateful for everything in my life. Each day is a gift because I came so close, so many times to not being here at all. I revel in each sunny day. I am joyful for the leaves turning in fall and for the blossoms of spring. I even stop these days in the middle of a thunderstorm, tilt my head up and feel the rain on my face. I catch snowflakes on my tongue. Sound trite? Maybe it is, but that's honestly how I feel. Not every day, all day, mind you. I still get frustrated, tired and down like everyone else, but I pull myself out quickly and remember what I have to be thankful for.

"Secondly, I am grateful for the people who love me. I am so incredibly fortunate. You know the saying, 'Laugh and the whole world laughs with you, cry and you cry alone.' I never experienced that. My family and friends stuck by me through the absolute worst. They fought for me, when there wasn't any hope left. They loved me, when I wasn't even me, only a shell that resembled my physical body was left behind. I will never be able to repay these people for what they gave me -- unconditional love. It's the greatest gift anyone can ever receive. You people know who you are. You are wonderful human beings. I love you.

"Also, there is something so liberating in finally understanding that as much as we would like to control our lives, as much as we would like to believe that we are the masters of our own destiny, we aren't. We can make our lists, run our errands, do our chores and pretend, but it can all be taken away in an instant. Everything can change in the blink of an eye. There is no control, so we'd better think twice when we decide to go to the grocery store instead of playing ball with our child. It may be the last opportunity we ever have to do it. I live my life much differently these days, because of that lesson. I try and squeeze as much life out of each and every day as I can. I give people the benefit of the doubt more often. I try and moderate my 'type A' tendencies. I tell my son, husband, mother, father, brother and everyone else who will listen how important they are to me. They probably get tired of hearing it, but I'll never stop.

"Finally and most importantly, I had to go through PPD to get my son, Zachary, and he was so worth it. I would go through it all again in a heartbeat for him, because he is my life, my love, my heart. I now know the secret that all parents do, I would give my life for his, in an instant, without even a second thought. It's a beautiful thing."

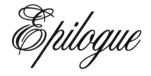

Epilogue

Update on Carolyn

Zachary is now two years old at this writing and Carolyn is fully recovered.

Carolyn and I collaborated on this book and we have worked hard together to get the book completed. She has been a tremendous help by setting up the interviews with various family members, reviewing the text, making sure of its accuracy and adding some of the emotional content. Carolyn, luckily, consulted with an old friend and mentor of hers who came up with the title for us. We love it! She was also instrumental in getting me into Mayo Clinic for the interviews.

She feels strongly that we need to get the word out about PPD, because no one really talks about it. The stigma attached to any type of mental illness keeps too many people from seeking treatment. Carolyn refuses to accept the stigma and has been courageous and steadfast throughout the book's

Mommies Cry Too

development.

Carolyn and her family, know, first-hand, how dangerous PPD can be and the effect it can have on a woman and her family. They also know how lucky they were to get through this and how close there were to not making it. They were on the "precipice."

There is no doubt that what got them through this were their loyal friends, but more importantly, the awesome strength of their family. In the struggle to get Carolyn back, her family pulled together and each one played his or her part. They relied on prayer, their strong will, hope, and the optimism that was part of all of them. Friends and family supported them when they could and sent a lot of prayers their way.

Will Carolyn have more children?

Carolyn's psychiatrist, whom she sees for medication on a regular basis, told her to find another way to add to their family other than giving birth. Carolyn commented with a twinkle in her eye, "I think he wants us to get a pet."

When Carolyn left Mayo Clinic she discussed with her

Mommies Cry Too

medical team the possibility of having another baby. She was told if she and Demain decided in the affirmative, they would need to plan carefully. A part of that plan would be if things started to go awry after the baby's birth, she would go to Mayo Clinic immediately and plan to stay for three weeks. And, they would get her back on track.

Grant Bauer, Carolyn's Clinical Social Worker at Mayo Clinic, says, "The Brinks are a very strong family and the key to success is knowing that Carolyn had this illness, and she can be treated and monitored by Mayo Clinic and the possibility of a positive outcome goes way up.

Dr. Clark is optimistic about a woman having a child after suffering from PPD. She said, "With a second birth, a woman and her partner know what to expect, there are usually fewer surprises. The key is careful planning during pregnancy with one's partner, therapist and psychiatrist for the needs of the woman and her family. Both emotional and instrumental support in the postpartum period are important. Requesting assistance from family members with whom there is not conflict or when affordable, hiring a person to help with cleaning, laundry, other household tasks and some childcare, can relieve some of the pressure for

140

both the woman and her partner.

Sounds like Good News!

What do Carolyn and Demian say? They wisely said, "We think the one thing this tale has taught us is that you never know what the future may hold and we are open to all possibilities."

Quote from Carolyn:
"If I had this to do all over again and I knew what I would have to go through, I would still have made the same decision to have a baby because: **Zachary was worth it all!"**

Family Pictures

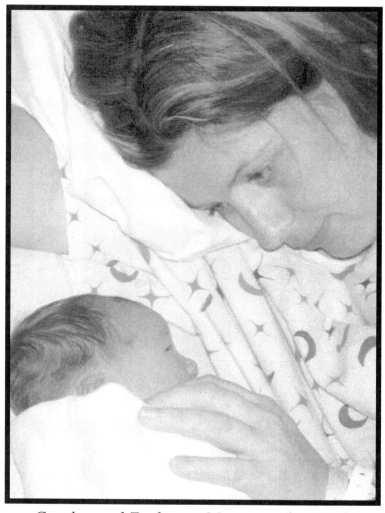

Carolyn and Zachary - Moments after Birth!

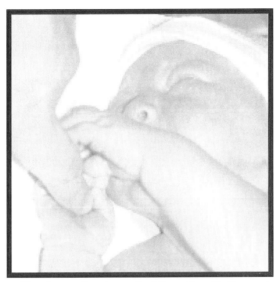

Newborn Zachary holding Dad's finger!

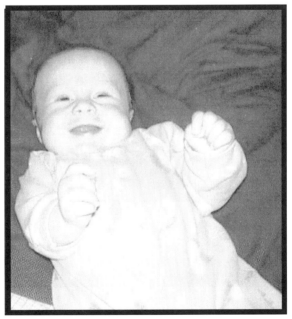

Baby Zachary

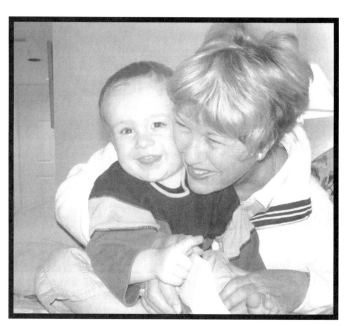

Grandma Mary-Jane & Zachary

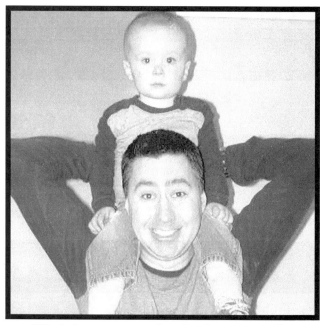

Who's having more fun, Zachary or Dad?

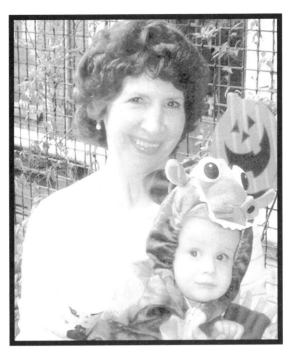

Zachary the frog with his "Guardian Angel", Betty

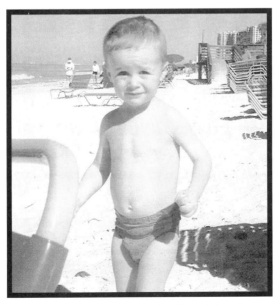

Zachary at the Beach!

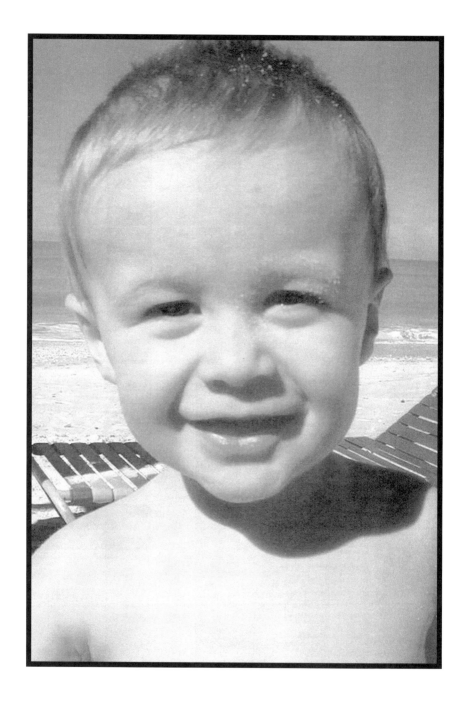

Zachary you're adorable. Mom was right you were worth it all!

The Keys to Carolyn's Survival

Her mother, Mary-Jane, who fortified by the tremendous love she had for her daughter, went through hell to bring her back from the brink of death. She used every resource available to her to find a solution.

Her husband, Demian, for his courage, and his never-wavering support and loyalty to Carolyn. His confidence in Mary-Jane, his mother-in-law, to make tough decisions and his flexibility to work together with her in finding a way to get Carolyn on the road to recovery.

Her father, Mike, who came on the scene at a critical juncture and made crucial decisions when Demian and Mary-Jane were emotionally exhausted.

Her brother and her extended family were there for her when she needed them.

Zachary's nanny, Betty, became a surrogate mom to Carolyn and Zachary. She had tremendous courage to try to help someone with PPD, an illness she knew very little about. She managed to infuse a spirit of <u>hope</u> where there was little left. She was critical to Carolyn's recovery.

Carolyn, herself, survived because of her indomitable will, determined nature and her analytical mind that was able, even in the depths of severe depression and extreme anxiety, to analyze her feelings and communicate her thoughts.

Carolyn survived because of her wonderful family. They all cared enough to fight for her and bring her back to health. And she made it all the way home.

Mayo Clinic, Carolyn and her family believe, saved her life. The CBTs helped tremendously to return her to a normal functioning person, but also the kindness, professionalism and hope the medical team gave her were so important to her complete recovery. She will always be indebted to all who helped her return to her family -- whole once again!

Note from the Author: Following Zachary's birth, the pediatrician discovered, what appeared to be at the time, a small and insignificant birth defect affecting his frenulum. This birth defect causes the tissue that attaches the tongue to the bottom of the mouth to be abnormally short (commonly known as tongue-tie). The tissue was clipped by the pediatrician.

If the frenulum is not corrected properly, it can cause feeding problems because the baby cannot latch onto the breast or even handle a bottle very well. The rejection of the breast, in retrospect, could have been caused by his seemingly inconsequential birth defect and his subsequent feeding problems. (When Zachary was sixteen months old it was discovered that the frenulum had grown back and needed to be corrected so Zachary was operated on for that correction.)

You cannot help but wonder if it was possible that the initial correction was not complete or that the frenulum grew back sooner, and if that had been discovered, maybe some of this agony could have been avoided. We will never know.

If you answered "yes" to 3 or more of the following symptoms, you may have postpartum depression. Call your doctor, and get professional help.

- sad or depressed mood
- loss of interest in things you used to enjoy
- feelings of guilt or hopelessness
- trouble concentrating or making decisions
- irritability or restlessness
- loss of energy
- sleep problems
- decreased or increased appetite
- weight loss or gain
- feeling overwhelmed
- worries/concerns about your ability to care for your baby
- not feeling close to/having difficulty bonding with your baby
- thoughts of harming yourself or your baby

Are you, or anyone you love, or know currently, experiencing any of the above symptoms?

Postpartum Treatment Program, University of Wisconsin, Psychiatric Clinic.

Comments from the Author

Carolyn's story was both a privilege and an agony to write. Strangely enough, the story is not really told by her but by the people closest to her because Carolyn lost her memory for three to four months following her son's birth. Her mother, husband, nanny and her best friend were all interviewed by me, along with her two psychiatrists and her social worker at Mayo Clinic. They tell Carolyn's story for her. Since Carolyn has such a dynamic personality, her presence is deeply felt in each person's description of her. When I interviewed Carolyn, she was frustrated that she could not contribute more to her story because she remembers very little of it. She obviously could tell me about her long recovery, and when her memory began to return. It was hard for me to imagine how difficult this experience must be because the memory loss includes the birth of her first child and the first three to four months of his life.

Why doesn't Carolyn remember? No one seems to be able to answer that completely. Some doctors say she may eventually remember. But most think the story is so painful it's probably best she doesn't remember and it's her mind's way of protecting her from further pain. She has come to terms with this memory loss and accepts it.

The most shocking part of this story is that Carolyn's mother and husband noticed, almost immediately after Zachary's birth, that something was wrong and got her medical care in less than two weeks. The diagnosis of PPD was made at this time. The frightening reality is that none of the usual treatments worked for her, like medication and therapy; in fact, her condition became worse, not better. She was treatment-resistant to severe depression, unfortunately, like over four million Americans are. As a last resort she was given ECT treatments, which usually work, but they did not appear to work for Carolyn. In desperation they went to Mayo Clinic and her life was saved. It was really a miracle. Carolyn's very strong personality helped that miracle to occur and her indomitable will pulled her out of the abyss of PPD.

Everyone I spoke with who knew Carolyn before her PPD "drew a picture" of a person I really wanted to know. Before writing this book, I barely knew Carolyn; I had met her very briefly when she was a college student. The next time I saw her was when she returned home from Mayo Clinic. Today I know her as the person whom everyone described to me, except that some of her stronger personality traits are tempered a bit and, as she says, she's mellowed some and wants to keep it that way.

Carolyn's courage to share her story with the public, despite the stigma that surrounds PPD, is admirable. I am honored to help in that endeavor by writing her story, about this period of her life, as told to me by her family, friends, and doctors.

References

Clark, Roseanne, Ph.D., *Mothers, Babies, and Depression*, 2001, University of Wisconsin Medical School

Chaudron, Linda H. M.D., M.S., *Postpartum Depression*, Pediatrics in Review, 2003, American Academy of Pediatrics

Chaudron, Linda, *Facts of Life*, Vol. 9, No. 11, 2004, Health Behavior News Service.

Frank, Jerome D. & Julia B., *Persuasion & Healing*, 1993 Johns Hopkins University Press, Baltimore and London

Mayo Clinic, *Cognitive Behavioral Therapy*, Mayo Foundation for Medical Education and Research

Mayo Clinic, Psychiatry & Psychology, *Mood Disorders Unit*, Mayo Foundation for Medical Education and Research

Mayo Clinic, *Understanding the Cytochrome P450 Test*, Mayo Foundation for Medical Education and Research

Mayo Clinic, *Understanding Antidepressant Medications,* Mayo Foundation for Medical Education and Research

Mayo Clinic, *Understanding Depression*, Mayo Foundation for Medical Education and Research

O'Hara, Michael, Chap. 3, *Portpartum Depression and Child Development,* 1997, The Guilford Press, New York and London

Osmond, Marie, *Behind the Smile*, Warner Books, New York

Padesky, Christine A., Greenberger, Dennis, *Clinician's Guide to Mind Over Mood*, 1995 The Guilford Press, New York, London

Shields, Brooke, *Down Came the Rain*, 2005 Hyperion, New York

We ask whoever reads this book to recommend it to another person so that we can spread the word about Postpartum Depression. Thank you for your help!

We are making 100 books available at _no charge_ on a first-request and need basis.
To make a request for a free book email us at: hartingtonpress@aol.com

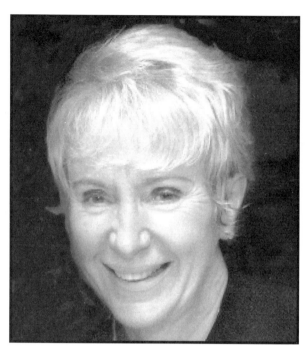

Carol S. Harcarik
Author of
"Mommies Cry Too"

Carol is an author and graphics designer.
She owns and operates her own publishing house, Hartington Press.
She was an English and Journalism major at
Douglas College for Women, Rutgers University.
She has written extensively for various newspapers and wrote her
father's memoirs and a historical book on one-room schoolhouses.
This is her largest journalistic project thus far
and she expects to do many more.

Hartington Press™